DEMANDING PATIENTS?

STATE OF HEALTH SERIES

Edited by Chris Ham, Director of Health Services Management Centre, University of Birmingham

DEMANDING PATIENTS?
Analysing the Use of
Primary Care

**Anne Rogers, Karen Hassell
and Gerry Nicolaas**

Open University Press
Buckingham · Philadelphia

Open University Press
Celtic Court
22 Ballmoor
Buckingham
MK18 1XW

email: enquiries@openup.co.uk
world wide web: http://www.openup.co.uk

and
325 Chestnut Street
Philadelphia, PA 19106, USA

First Published 1999

A catalogue record of this book is available from the British Library

ISBN   0 335 20091 5 (hb)   0 335 20090 7 (pb)

Library of Congress Cataloging-in-Publication Data
Rogers, Anne.
    Demanding patients?: analysing the use of primary care/Anne
Rogers, Karen Hassell, Gerry Nicolaas.
    p. cm. – (State of health series)
    Includes bibliographical references and index.
    ISBN 0-335-20090-7 (pb)
    [DNLM: 1. National Health Service (Great Britain) 2. Primary
Health Care – Utilization – Great Britain. 3. Patient Acceptance of
Health Care. 4. Health Services Needs and Demand – Great Britain.
5. Self Care – Utilization – Great Britain. 6. State Medicine –
organization & administration – Great Britain. W 84.6 R724d 1998]
RA399.G7R65   1998
DNLM/DLC
for Library of Congress   98–4299
                                                               CIP

Typeset by Type Study, Scarborough
Printed in Great Britain by St Edmundsbury Press, Bury St Edmunds

CONTENTS

Part III: Mediating demand in primary care

SERIES EDITOR'S INTRODUCTION

Health services in many developed countries have come under critical scrutiny in recent years. In part this is because of increasing expenditure, much of it funded from public sources, and the pressure this has put on governments seeking to control public spending. Also important has been the perception that resources allocated to health services are not always deployed in an optimal fashion. Thus at a time when the scope for increasing expenditure is extremely limited, there is a need to search for ways of using existing budgets more efficiently. A further concern has been the desire to ensure access to health care of various groups on an equitable basis. In some countries this has been linked to a wish to enhance patient choice and to make service providers more responsive to patients as 'consumers'.

Underlying these specific concerns are a number of more fundamental developments which have a significant bearing on the performance of health services. Three are worth highlighting. First, there are demographic changes, including the ageing population and the decline in the proportion of the population of working age. These changes will both increase the demand for health care and at the same time limit the ability of health services to respond to this demand.

Second, advances in medical science will also give rise to new demands within the health services. These advances cover a range of possibilities, including innovations in surgery, drug therapy, screening and diagnosis. The pace of innovation is likely to quicken as the end of the century approaches, with significant implications for the funding and provision of services.

Third, public expectations of health services are rising as those who use services demand higher standards of care. In part, this is stimulated by developments within the health service, including the availability of new technology. More fundamentally, it stems from the emergence of a more educated and informed population, in which people are accustomed to being treated as consumers rather than patients.

Against this background, policymakers in a number of countries are reviewing the future of health services. Those countries which have traditionally relied on a market in health care are making greater use of regulation and planning. Equally, those countries which have traditionally relied on regulation and planning are moving towards a more competitive approach. In no country is there complete satisfaction with existing methods of financing and delivery, and everywhere there is a search for new policy instruments.

The aim of this series is to contribute to debate about the future of health services through an analysis of major issues in health policy. These issues have been chosen because they are both of current interest and of enduring importance. The series is intended to be accessible to students and informed lay readers as well as to specialists working in this field. The aim is to go beyond a textbook approach to health policy analysis and to encourage authors to move debate about their issue forward. In this sense, each book presents a summary of current research and thinking, and an exploration of future policy directions.

Professor Chris Ham
Director of Health Services Management Centre,
University of Birmingham

ACKNOWLEDGEMENTS

Many people have contributed to the writing of this book. This includes a number of our colleagues at the National Primary Care Research and Development Centre who have been a rich source of ideas and have discussed the issues with us at various points in its preparation. We are particularly grateful for the research input provided by Alison Chapple, Leslie Hallam, Shirley Halliwell and Michelle Sergison. We are also grateful to Heather Eliott and Steve Rose for searching databases and collecting and collating abstracts and articles which we have used in some of our analysis. Thanks too are due to Gill Geraghty and Margarita Cook for help with the bibliography. As well as our colleagues we are grateful to a number of other people who have contributed to the ideas we have drawn upon. In discussing and debating the issues of the management of demand we have drawn heavily upon the ideas of Philip Hadridge (Anglia and Oxford NHSE), David Pencheon (Institute of Public Health, University of Cambridge) and Vikki Entwistle (Centre for Reviews and Dissemination, University of York). The Access to Care Reference Group set up by Oxford and Anglia NHSE has also provided a stimulating forum for the discussion of ideas which informed the analysis presented here. Finally we are grateful to David Pilgrim who has provided invaluable sociological insights and helped considerably with editing.

Anne Rogers
Karen Hassell
Gerry Nicolaas

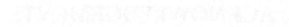

INTRODUCTION

A defining feature of health and welfare services in advanced capitalist societies is their inability to meet the aspirations and expectations of significant groups in the population. The demand for public and private utility services outweighs the capacity to supply them and some people are unable to get the services they want and need. Methods for containing cost and increasingly sophisticated consumer demands are exhausting traditional service responses. Decreasing economic growth and the capacity of advanced welfare states to meet existing commitments to health and welfare are likely to exacerbate the problem.

Within the health care sector, managing the gap between the demand for health care and the ability to supply it is viewed as a major health policy challenge. Concern has been voiced by professionals and policy makers about the pressure of burgeoning workloads and the increasing 'expectations' of the population for health care. Tension between the demand for health services and the cost of providing them has led health care systems to adopt explicit or implicit rationing strategies. In the British National Health Service (NHS) this has been brought to the fore by quasi-markets separating purchasing from providing activities (Mechanic 1995). Alongside concerns to manage the scale of demand for health services, there has been a parallel desire to meet unmet need and reduce inequalities in health care and health status. There is recognition that an undue emphasis on trying to control or diminish demand could deflect attention from underuse among certain groups in the population (DoH 1996).

The need to manage demand within the NHS threatens the basic social contract set up between the public and the state in its original aim of providing a service free at the point of need. Since its inception there has been ambiguity over whether or not the NHS should and could meet all of the demands for health care of a population. The meeting of need by the NHS was originally viewed as fundamental to ensuring a reduction in the demand for services. The Beveridge Report noted the presence of an 'untreated pool of illness' which would have to be dealt with. Once this had happened it was assumed that demand would stabilize at a lower level. However, the possibility that demand for health services would always outstrip supply was also evident from the outset. Not only did some of Bevan's contemporaries warn that it was wrong to assume that demand for health care was finite (Allsop 1994) but in a speech just before the NHS was established in 1948, Bevan commented that:

> We never will have all we need. Expectation will always exceed capacity. This service must always be changing, growing and improving, it must always appear inadequate.
>
> (Foot 1975: 209–10)

Concerns with 'health need' inside the NHS have grown since the late 1980s when the government required health authorities to assess the needs of local populations (Seedhouse 1994). The needs assessment industry in health services research has also burgeoned over the last decade. Despite this increased focus on needs there has been far less emphasis on understanding and responding to the gap between need and demand. In particular, there has been a failure to explore in depth the relationship between need, demand and the supply of services from the point of view of an understanding of patient action and views. Instead the discourse on demand tends to focus on the concept of 'expectations' as an explanatory factor in accounting for rising demand. The term 'expectation' when associated with the cause of demand carries with it connotations of excessiveness or irrationality. For example, Levitt and Wall (1991) distinguish between 'need based on an objective assessment against known criteria' and 'demand on the other hand, (which) is more volatile and is based on expectations, realistic or not'. 'Demand' conjures up a view of people using health care as petulant children demanding what cannot realistically be provided by overworked professionals in a hard-pressed health service. The discourse of 'expectations' when discussed in relation to 'demand' is one-sided and tends to ignore the fact that the public's responsibility around providing health care and maintaining health has *increased* in recent years. (Witness, for example, the growing popularity of the adoption of healthier lifestyles, the push towards home births and campaigns to demedicalize disability and mental health problems as a means of lay people taking control and responsibility for their own health.) Nor from this vantage point are the diversity, complexity and gene- sis of expectations among different population groups subjected to detailed examination or viewed as subject to change by the par- ameters of our medical and health institutions and professions. Most importantly, focusing crudely on 'expectation' deflects us from a wider exploration of people's actions and the way in which they seek out formal health care, opt for inaction, or rely on informal care and self-care in preference to using services. It is the latter which form the focus of our analysis in this book.

A number of interfaces are implicated in understanding and responding to demand in the health service. These include the interface between and within formally provided health service sec- tors: e.g. within and between primary and secondary care, health and social care. Recent government policies flag up the importance of a multi-sectoral approach in tackling inequalities in health prob- lems and responding to ill health. The recent public health policy *Our Healthier Nation* gives prominence to a three-tiered approach in bringing about change. This includes action taken at the levels of government and national players, locality and community and by individuals. Our analysis in this book focuses on the interface between lay and formal health care, particularly primary care. The primary care focus reflects its gatekeeping role and its importance in recent British health policy. Primary care is the point in the system which is influenced by patients' decision making about when and how to access services. Only a small proportion of health care problems are seen in primary care. So, small changes in the behav- iour of the population, or in the accessibility and organization of a service, could produce large changes in the demand for formal care. The concept of primary care is used in two ways in this book. It is used in its more traditional sense of defining primary care as con- stituted by the organizational aspects of formal service provision. This includes general practice and primary health care teams with pharmacy and other practitioners operating at the periphery. It also considers primary care as the utilization of all of the various sources of care available to respond to new illness episodes. This includes the less visible self-care and informal primary care provided by non-professionals. It also refers to alternative sources of care such as osteopathy, homeopathy and other forms of complementary practice when used as a supplement to or substitute for the formal primary care services.

Exploring the relationship between health need and demand for care is not new. Its importance was identified in the concept of 'illness behaviour' more than 35 years ago by Mechanic who pointed out that:

> the realm of illness behaviour falls logically and chronologically between the two major concerns of medical science etiology and therapy. Variables affecting illness behaviour come into play prior to medical scrutiny and treatment but after etiological processes have been initiated. In this sense illness behaviour events determine whether diagnosis and treatment will begin at all.
>
> (Mechanic 1961)

Since that time a wealth of sociological literature focusing on the meaning and actions that people take in responding to health and illness has extended our knowledge and understanding of lay meanings and responses to health and illness. As a result, our understanding of illness behaviour has increased significantly over the last 20 years. The point here is not to replicate what has already been well researched elsewhere. Instead we will draw on this rich body of existing knowledge together with our own primary research in providing a contemporary analysis of need, demand and help seeking at the interface between lay and formal care.

This book examines the patterns and social processes influencing the use of formal care; the relationship between people's conceptions and experience of illness; self-management and informal management of illness; and their use of formal services. These relate to a number of facets of the relationship between the health care sector and the populations they serve including locality, family, economic and social resources and personal health biographies of people using services. We draw on exemplars, and messages from two areas of research carried out at the National Primary Care Research and Development Centre. These include a qualitative and quantitative study of pathways to care and an ethnographic study of advice giving in pharmacy. Further details of these projects are provided in the Appendix.

In Chapter 1 we examine the way in which need and demand have been conceptualized in the context of the NHS. Our starting premise is that definitions and approaches to the understanding of health need, demand and use of services are complex and contested. We are concerned with illustrating the way in which definitions of need and demand are problematic because it is possible to contest them conceptually and define them contingently. Clinical models of need are the basis of the new trend towards evidence-based practice, the goal of which will be to target effective services and interventions in a way which maps onto the need for health care. The issue of health, need and demand involves the making of value judgements. What comes to be seen as appropriate or inappropriate demand is shaped by the activities and interests of parties or stakeholders within the NHS. The different ways of managing demand are also explored. We point to the way a deficiency has arisen in excluding an in-depth understanding and involvement of lay people in responding to the problem of the demand for health care.

The construction of the problem of inappropriate demand in primary care forms the focus of Chapter 2. We describe the way in which a 'patient defect' model has dominated the notion of inappropriate demand within formal primary care. Such a view has become detached from evidence of the impact that organizational arrangements, professional behaviour and changing working practices have had on creating and shaping demand. Moreover, the patient 'defect' model tends to be ignorant of what patients themselves consider to be appropriate and inappropriate demand.

The focus of Chapter 3 shifts to the approaches which have been deployed to understand influences on help seeking and entry into the health care system. The focus on symptoms as the main explanatory factor in consulting behaviour has a number of limitations. We describe these as a backdrop to examining the characteristics of the traditional health utilization models, including the health belief, rational choice and socio-behavioural approaches, and discuss their strengths and weaknesses. The social process approach is assessed in terms of its ability to understand the process of decision making and the outcome of help seeking as a product of the interaction of people with others and of other factors which are often beyond an individual's control.

In Chapter 4 we explore the way in which the experience of illness and service use shapes people's help seeking. We draw on our own qualitative research on 'pathways to care' to illustrate the process of the lay evaluation of illness, and the relationship between past and future use of services. We continue in Chapter 5 by presenting data which illustrate the different patterns of help seeking used by people in accessing contemporary primary care services. We also explore the parameters of, and contingencies related to, the containment of illness and triggers to seek care. We move on to examine the influence of people's social networks in mediating the demand for formal care.

In Chapter 6 we examine the way in which people act as providers of primary care, the sources and nature of informal and self-care and the relevance of these within the context of developing a demand management strategy at the interface between lay and primary care. Using our own research data, we draw attention to the importance of interactions between doctors and patients in people's understanding of the legitimacy of self-care practices.

In Chapter 7 we turn our attention to the role of community pharmacy in mediating demand and reinforcing patients' own self-care actions. We highlight the importance of analysing the use of pharmacists as an alternative to the GP and as a resource for self-care, the role of pharmacists as agents of referral to GPs and the importance of locality in shaping the nature of advice which is provided by pharmacies to the public.

The development of relevant and meaningful information is increasingly being seen as an important aspect of improving demand management. Consequently, in Chapter 8 the role of information is analysed critically in relation to informed decision making, self-care and demand management strategies. As well as the impact of official information, we also look at the way in which diverse unofficial sources of information impact on people's decision making in accessing primary care services.

In the final chapter we turn our attention to the policy implications which arise out of our analysis of primary care use. We argue for an approach which changes the culture of the delivery of services to one which involves patients and professionals operating as partners in health care decisions.

PART I

POLICY CONTEXT, INFLUENCES AND APPROACHES TO UNDERSTANDING DEMAND AND USE OF SERVICES

1

CONCEPTUALIZING NEED AND DEMAND IN THE NHS

Within modern health systems, clients by definition do not know exactly what they demand because the supply side itself defines the treatment required by clients.

(C. Offe, *Contradictions of the Welfare State*)

There are few presumptions in human relations more dangerous than the idea that one knows what another human being needs better than they do themselves.

(Michael Ignatieff, *The Needs of Strangers*)

The Introduction has noted the problems created for modern health and welfare systems by the increasing demand for services. In Britain the NHS has found it difficult to sustain its founding social contract of providing services free at the point of need. Managing demand and ensuring access to services for patients remain central challenges for policy makers. An understanding of the various aspects of the demand for, need for, and use of contemporary health care is, of necessity, highly complex. It requires an in-depth analysis of processes within and outside the NHS.

In this book our particular interest within this complexity is on the actions and views of lay people in their management of illness and their use of primary care. There is a particular focus on the use of primary care because of its gatekeeping role and the importance attributed to it in recent British health policy. It is the point in the system which is most influenced by patients' decision making about when and how to access services. It is also the closest NHS interface with the responses to illness episodes provided by people outside formal care.

   This first chapter will critically analyse the policy context of, and relationship between:

- need,
- demand (as the expression of want or need),
- supply (those health facilities available to provide care),
- approaches to the management of the latter.

In conceptualizing the relationship between need and demand, various definitions in common currency are analysed. The methods of demand management that have been or are being considered as having relevance for the NHS will be explored. In the final section we highlight the relevance of focusing on the actions of ordinary people in mapping the complexities of health services use in primary care.

NEED AND DEMAND IN THE CONTEXT OF CONTEMPORARY HEALTH POLICY

Need is a complex and contested notion which rarely surfaces in analyses of demand for services. This disjuncture between need and use of services is evident at the levels of health research and policy making. For example, research on health inequalities has focused on either the economic and social determinants of the health status of population groups, *or* the distribution, availability, and access to health services. Despite evidence that people in disadvantaged groups not only have higher mortality rates and experience increased morbidity but are also less likely to receive good health care (Ben-Shlomo and Chaturvedi 1995), most analyses of health care and their management within primary care have continued to focus either on epidemiology or on illnesses being presented in general practice, with relatively little attention paid to processes, such as 'access' which connects the two.

Perspectives and interests in defining need

In recent years a significant contribution has been made by moral philosophy to the conceptualization of human needs, in distinguishing between 'need', 'desire' and 'interest' and in clarifying the distinction between 'fundamental' or 'categorical' need and 'relative' need. For our purposes, when examining the *use* of health services, we are mainly interested in the need and demand *for care* rather than 'health need' *per se*.[1] In developing a stakeholder perspective on need, Williams (1983) points to the coexistence of different interests in the process of need definition within a policy context. In her scheme, the construction of need involves both dominant professional and subordinate patient interests. These may be synergistic (i.e. they converge) or non-synergistic (i.e. they are discrepant). Separating out differing perspectives is necessarily an interpretive task. Positions are not always clearly defined or consciously adopted. Views on 'appropriateness' may be held at a collective professional level as well as at the individual practitioner level and may be more deeply embedded in some professional cultures, such as bio-medicine, than in others. Notions of need also change according to the immediate health policy context. For example, the 1990s reforms have incorporated contracting for services as a key feature of a quasi-market system. This contract culture has been associated with needs assessment activities as part of targeting the improvement of quality and effectiveness, the rationing of health care and other courses of action taken by health authorities. As Sheaff (1996) has commented:

> Health service managers are increasingly joining clinicians and other health workers in using the language of needs to justify local changes in health services – changes that typically redefine what health care will be available and often ration access to it . . .
>
> (Sheaff 1996: 1)

Notwithstanding the recent impact of managerialism on needs assessment activities, the notion of 'clinically defined need' retains its dominance in health services policy making and practice. 'Clinical need' defined as the need for medical services is the basis on which the NHS was established. Despite the rise in the popularity of other definitions and portmanteau models, it continues to have the greatest salience. Briefly stated, the clinical perspective is predicated either on an epidemiological/symptom-based definition (such as the level and type of symptoms in the community – see Chapter 3) or on one defined by symptoms or signs for which there is an 'effective' ameliorative or curative intervention. Within evidence-based medicine (EBM), which has considerable currency in contemporary health policy making, need is often translated into whether a condition can be treated with available knowledge, technology and resources, in order

to ensure that decisions about the provision and delivery of
clinical services are driven increasingly by evidence of clinical
and cost effectiveness coupled with the systematic assessment
of health outcomes.

(NHS Executive 1996: 6)

Perspectives from within the social sciences provide a different
orientation towards health need. These pay attention to the social
factors and contexts which influence the formulation of need in
relation to the use of services. Some social science definitions do
incorporate absolute notions of health need, which are not dissimi-
lar from clinical perspectives. For example, Doyal and Gough
(1991) adopt a categorical notion of physical impairment as the
basis for assessing health. The Doyal and Gough approach can be
distinguished from a more dominant social science, one which
emphasizes the relative nature of need, with the latter being socially
constructed. This starts from the premise that an individual sufferer's needs may be constructed by the extent to which symptoms
disrupt everyday activities and the extent to which they are fearful
or embarrassing. By contrast, for close relatives, need may reflect
behaviour which is unwanted or disruptive to family functioning
(Clausen and Yarrow 1955; Oliver 1990). Social science notions of
need also highlight the importance of quality of life, the absence of
well-being and the role of socio-economic and structural factors.
Greater weight is attributed to the experience of illness through
self-reports and to socio-economic factors and definitions of need
from users themselves (Fitzpatrick *et al.* 1986). This approach has
also tended to contrast subjective definitions of health problems
with clinical representations of need. This is evident in Oliver's consideration of disability:

> The social world differs from the natural world in (at least) one
> fundamental respect; that is, human beings give meanings to
> objects in the social world and subsequently orientate their
> behaviour to these objects in terms of the meanings given to
> them. W.I. Thomas succinctly puts it thus: 'if men [*sic*] define
> situations as real, they are real in their consequences'. As far as
> disability is concerned, if it is seen as a tragedy, then disabled
> people will be treated as if they are the victims of some tragic
> happening or circumstance ... Alternatively, it logically fol-
> lows that if disability is defined as social oppression, then
> disabled people will be seen as the collective victims of an
> uncaring or unknowing society rather than as individual

victims of circumstance. Such a view will be translated into social policies geared towards alleviating oppression rather than compensating individuals.

(Oliver 1990: 2/3)

Social science approaches have also inclined to be explicitly normative in their analyses of need. They have prioritized political, social and economic factors affecting need rather than the diagnostic signs and symptoms focus of a clinical approach to need[2] (Bradshaw 1972).

These broad distinctions between clinical and social formulations of need sometimes break down or become blurred. For example, the work of Doyal and Gough has been cited. In the other direction, some clinical approaches to defining need now adopt concepts from within the social sciences. A large number of clinical studies now combine morbidity with other information and perspectives.[3] Also multidimensional notions of the need for services have become more popular with the recognition of the shortcomings of unidimensional measures of need. A recognition of different versions of health need have been incorporated and developed into typologies of need. For example, Bradshaw (1972) distinguishes between four types of need which have been widely used and developed in applied research in the health and social care field.

1 *Normative* need is that which is defined by experts and professionals. Within a health context this involves need being mainly defined by medical norms and clinical standards and criteria (e.g. the absence or presence of signs and symptoms of disease).
2 *Felt* need relates to wants or desires. In relation to health and illness this relates to the subjective experience of health.
3 *Expressed* need is felt need transformed into action. In the case of demand for primary care, for example, this relates to the proportion of illness which is presented to formal services.
4 *Comparative* need within a health context relates to equity and the impact of disadvantage and inequalities on need.

Bradshaw's distinctions are useful, not only because they solve unending debates about how to define needs but also how to respond to them. The distinctions highlight the potential tensions which exist among the four categories, and suggest that services designed to respond mainly to one type of need may fail to address another defined in a different way.

The problem of demand

Demand is most frequently understood to mean the expression of need among population groups. As we mentioned in the Introduction, it can carry negative connotations of excessiveness. Unlike 'need' (a subjective psychological or philosophical notion), demand and supply are objectivist concepts borrowed from economics. Supply refers to the quantity of a commodity that providers are willing to offer for sale at a price. Demand refers to the quantity of the commodity that consumers are prepared to buy at a specified price. Although there is an assumed relationship between demand and need, this tends to be poorly operationalized and rarely the subject of exploration.[4] In relation to health care, the supply side defines need, tautologically, as a problem for which there is an intervention that is 'effective'.[5] As a result, the complexities of the need for health care have remained relatively separate from discussions about demand.

Pencheon (1996) identifies three dimensions of demand which conjecture a relationship of dependence and interdependence with services. The assumption of the relationship between service user and supplier in relation to the three dimensions is as follows:

- *Demand for interventions.* Increased medical technology and ability to screen, diagnose and treat illness has created a technological imperative to seek care. This is similar to Illich's notion of cultural iatrogenesis: 'medical practice sponsors sickness by reinforcing a morbid society' (Illich 1976: 35), which encourages people to become consumers of curative medicine and health services.
- *Demand for convenience and quality.* Consumerism has led to greater expectations from public services such as the NHS. A demand for quality, a sensitivity to idiosyncratically expressed needs, and an expectation of personal convenience have all become part of a new consumerism.
- *Demand for meaningful involvement* has also been part of the philosophy of recent planning and services provision. Service user groups and service commissioners have demanded or encouraged user involvement at both the collective level and at the level of the individual patient's partnership with professionals offering him or her care.

Discussions of policy makers and managers of the NHS have centred on the extent[6] and appropriateness of demand and the means of managing these. In describing the range of likely reasons for an increase of pressures on health systems caused by demand, Pencheon (1996) distinguishes between population changes and changes in clinical practice as follows.

Population changes

- Increased public expectation from a more informed, prosperous and empowered public (e.g. health products as items of consumption); changing norms in services industry (e.g. 24-hour financial services).
- Increased relative social deprivation.
- Changes in health behaviour (e.g. drug misuse).
- Increased demand for meeting chronic health needs.
- Demographic changes (e.g. an ageing population).
- Increases in the incidence of disease.
- Changes in patterns of disease (e.g. HIV, chronic fatigue syndrome).

Changes in clinical practice

- Increased diagnostic technology leading to increased disease detection rates.
- Increased therapeutic technology (e.g. treatment of cataracts and coronary artery bypass grafts).
- Multiple admissions related to decreased length of hospital stays (e.g. 'revolving door' patients in acute psychiatric services).
- Professional desire to offer the best possible care.
- Decreased referral threshold (e.g. from primary to secondary care).
- Fears of litigation increases referral rates and the need to intervene.

The list of likely reasons is schematic at present, with more being known about some items than others. For example, taking the first item in the first list above, little is known about which cohorts in the population are 'informed, prosperous and empowered' and how the processes which increase public expectations translate into demand for more services. Similarly, with regard to the contribution of the changing incidence and patterns of disease, there is evidence, for example, of rising morbidity in relation to childhood asthma, nocturnal asthma symptoms in adults and self-poisoning (Capewell 1996; Kendrick 1996). However, these occasional increases in recorded morbidity cannot account for the scale of rising demand. Some commentators have in fact pointed out that there is little to suggest major changes in the incidence of most diseases (NAHAT 1994). Neither, does it seem, do demographic changes account for the large increases in demand for services seen in recent years. For example, it has been estimated that only 2 per cent of the increase in emergency hospital admissions in Scotland and England can be accounted for by older people (NAHAT 1994; Kendrick 1996). There has been increased demand in all age and diagnostic groups (though there is evidence that this is skewed towards socially deprived groups; see Black 1993). While each of the items in Pencheon's list may be plausible hypotheses, the way they might interact and the extent of their relative contribution to increased demand about a particular type of problem remains unknown.

Appropriate and inappropriate demand

Like need, the problem of what constitutes rising or appropriate demand is also socially constructed. For example, the policy environment can shape the parameters of this problem. Demand for primary care out of hours, for example, is viewed as a growing problem in the UK but does not appear to be viewed in this way in France. This may in part be related to the system of remuneration in the French health care system, where out-of-hours calls are undertaken by junior doctors, costing the state less than consultations with more senior medical practitioners during the day.

As with the concept of need, there are various lay, policy and professional interests and meanings attached to the notions of 'appropriate' and 'inappropriate' demand. Operationalizing a definition of what constitutes appropriate demand at an individual level is fraught with problems. Judgements using symptoms as the basis for attributions of appropriateness can only be made with the wisdom of hindsight and the nature of illness is such that symptoms remain uncertain for diagnosing physicians as well as for lay people (Field 1976; Green and Dale 1992). Additionally, as we examine in the next chapter, rather than being fixed and predetermined, notions of appropriateness are often part of a *negotiated* process at the level of doctor and patient interaction (Punamaki and Kokko 1995b).

The construction of appropriate demand for treatment and care also occurs at the boundaries between primary and secondary care and between different specialties within the NHS. Physicians and surgeons may view the presentation for treatment of a person with

'Munchausen Syndrome' as an unwarranted use of health service resources. By contrast, a psychiatrist or psychologist might view the patient's underlying psychological state as the legitimate presentation of the need for 'treatment'. Similarly, what is considered to be appropriate demand according to standard medical criteria in general practice may be less certain than hospital-based specialty criteria. For example, there is some evidence to suggest that specialists' and GPs' criteria of appropriate referral are different. In relation to depression, specialists consider that GPs under-diagnose and under-treat (Armstrong *et al.* 1991). Adherence to EBM criteria may also turn some conditions previously considered appropriately dealt with by the NHS into inappropriate demand. These differences are shaped both by differences in the socialization of clinical sub-specialties and by the various work contexts within the health service.

There are also differences between providers and users as to what may constitute appropriate demand. For example, public health physicians are frequently credited with being sympathetic to lay conceptions of health need in health gain strategies, and they are likely to view the heavy use of services as being located within a health care system which does not pay sufficient attention to environmental and social reform (Malone 1995). However, in the case of immunization 'uptake', they still have a tendency at times to override parental preferences when pursing a collective population interest (Rogers and Pilgrim 1995). There is also evidence of differences in the formulation of type of demand between patient groups and provider criteria. The waiting lists for standard surgical procedures such as hip replacement may be growing, but so is the rising popularity of alternative therapies based on a rejection of conventional medicines. Not only do services fail to meet some types of need, but in some instances they may sustain the provision of inappropriate care when meeting demand with iatrogenic or ineffective services. The provision of inappropriate services and calls for non-intervention among certain patient groups also amount to a rejection of the supply available to meet demand. (An example of this is the unpopularity of conventional psychiatric interventions such as ECT and major tranquillizers among some mental health users.) Even where there is apparent mutual convergence of an interest in the personal experience and definition of needs from providers or commissioners, the volume of services available from the latter may fail to match the expressed needs of certain groups (Pilgrim *et al.* 1997).

DEMAND FOR FORMAL VERSUS INFORMAL CARE

Because of the focus on resources in health debates, demand is viewed almost exclusively in terms of the volume and effectiveness of formally provided health services. A focus on the demand for *existing services* rather than the demand for health care in general precludes the consideration of activity outside formally delivered services. Compared to formal services the informal health care system represents the 'black economy' of health care provision. For most of the time it remains invisible and excluded from the agendas of policy makers.

Aspects of formal services are mirrored in the demand for, and supply of, informal care. Both systems of care involve considerations of availability, rationing and scarcity. However, the type of need addressed by professionally delivered public services differs in some respects from that provided for by informal, familial or self-care. The state attempts to provide for physical and social need through formal welfare, health and social services. They provide care impersonally. The connection between the resourcing of services (the taxpayers) and the recipients of services (the patients) is severed by the organizational arrangements of the welfare state. Other needs cannot be provided for by the contemporary welfare state but are potentially met by informal, kin or friendship networks (Ignatieff 1994). For example, even though professional discourses use notions such as TLC, 'tender loving care', it is usually acknowledged that the basic human need to receive love cannot be met by health care professionals. The meeting of one set of needs by formal health services may give rise to others. Among older people, need for assistance with personalized activities for daily living, such as bathing, and need for instrumental activities, such as housework, takes away the value attached to another fundamental need: being self-sufficient and independent (Bury and Holmes 1990).

The distinction between informal and formal means of meeting need are not static. The boundaries between the two may become blurred or even reversed and may differ for various groups of people. In relation to those with severe mental health problems, for example, professionals have been found to provide the main social network contacts and to substitute the type of contact more usually provided by lay people (Estroff and Zimmer 1994; Spiker *et al.* 1995). In relation to 'simple' back pain evidence-based guidelines used in primary care advocate the use of self-care measures in preference to traditional bio-medical treatments (Roland and Dixon 1989). The importance of informal health care as a means of meeting demand is discussed further in Chapter 6.

THE MANAGEMENT OF DEMAND

The concept of demand management

At a policy level some coyness has traditionally accompanied discussions of demand management. The latter is associated with rationing which has encountered problems of legitimation from the public and professionals. However, managing demand better has been part of a changing language and ethos brought in by a quasi-marketized health care system (Mechanic 1995). While terms such as 'rationing' have been around for some time, formal definitions of managing demand have only recently begun to emerge within health debates. These emerging definitions place different emphases on the points at which demand might most effectively be managed. Some analysts target the need to modify or change individual patient behaviour. Vickery and Lynch (1995), for example, view demand management as supporting individuals in order that they can make 'rational' health and medical decisions based on the consideration of risks and benefits. Others have taken a broader systemic view. They link the management of demand to all parts of the health system, including the interfaces between the various parts (e.g. between primary and secondary care). This is evident in a definition espoused by Pencheon:

> demand management is the process of identifying where, how, why and by whom, demand for health care is made; and the best methods of curtailing, coping or creating this demand such that the most cost effective, appropriate, and equitable health care system can be developed. In short: how can supply and demand for health care be reconciled.
>
> (Pencheon 1996)

This view of the management of demand is seen as involving three interlinked elements:

- curtailing the demand for ineffective and the least cost-effective services,
- coping better with demand for effective services – changing the supply through 're-engineering',

- creating demand for services which are known to be cost-effective but are under-utilized by patients and under-deployed by professionals.

Implicit and explicit demand management strategies have manifested themselves either at the supply end of health care or at the level of modifying individuals' demand for health care. Overall, and most notable in Europe, there has been a greater focus on curtailing or managing the supply side. Demand management strategies have been most visible in marketized health care systems. In the United States, for example, demand management strategies have been closely associated with the introduction of 'managed care' in Health Maintenance Organizations. They were a direct response to the escalating costs and reducing profits of health insurance companies (Robinson and Steiner 1998). The tools of ' managed care' (Smith 1997) include:

- a capitation payment for every person for whom care is provided,
- gatekeepers, advice lines to patients,
- user fees for consumer education,
- medical management: including utilization review (doctors have to seek permission before referring patients or spending large amounts of money),
- pre-admission certification,
- disease management: greater use of guidelines, telemedicine (e.g. advice and consultation provided by a TV link or via the Internet and the World Wide Web) and non-doctors.

Similar demand management tools are being deployed in all systems of care and it has recently been commented upon that the NHS: 'is in many ways one giant managed care system' (Smith 1997). The formal tools of managed care are inextricably bound up with informal tools of managing demand. Higgins and Ruddell (1991) describe a list of 'seven Ds' – a mixture of overt and covert strategies of demand management within contemporary health services:

- *Don't tell* (not informing people of all available options/benefits and risks).
- *Demarket* (the discouragement of the use of services).
- *Deter* (making access difficult/inconvenient: the continuation of the inverse care law indicates the deterrence of use by shortage of supply).
- *Delay* (waiting lists).

- *Debate* (public relations encouraging more rational use of services).
- *Demarcate* (limiting the amount of any intervention in a quota).
- *Deny* (not offering a particular service).

The use of the 'D' word is also evident in a more recent analysis of responses to managing the gap between need and demand. Øvretveit (1997) points to ethical dilemmas associated with each of these.

- *Do nothing* (access becomes restricted through longer waiting lists: unethical due to increasing inequities in access and a drift towards private insurance).
- *Do more with the same or less resources* (through incentives, automation, stronger management and effectiveness: unethical when it results in exploitation of underpaid and junior staff).
- *Do more with more resources* (shifting the burden of care onto the unpaid work force and other parties such as employers, e.g. shortening hospital stays and employer-paid health insurance schemes: unethical as creates inequities in access and health status).
- *Define health needs more narrowly and change behaviour* (narrowing the definition of need to clinical need met by effective interventions: unethical as it disadvantages poor and vulnerable people most in need of health and social care).

Rationing

Modifying supply and rationing services have been the dominant ways of attempting to control demand within the NHS in the UK. 'Rationing' and 'prioritizing' have been defined by Øvretveit (1997) as follows:

> Rationing is restricting supply by explicit or implicit means, where demand exceeds supply, and where market mechanisms do not relate supply to demand in an acceptable way. Prioritising is deciding who goes first, or the relative proportion of resources allocated to a patient, patient group, population or service.
>
> (1997: 77)

Rationing strategies have been attempted at different levels. They range from transparent and planned mechanisms, to types of *ad hoc*, informal and covert mechanisms. These strategies operate at both the macro level of strategic planning, where attempts are made to operationalize general principles of rationing within trusts and commissioning organizations, and at the micro level of professional practice. Many health authorities now make explicit decisions not to offer certain services. This amounts to curtailing the demand for services by cutting off the supply. Some procedures, such as fertility treatment, the removal of tattoos, and sterilization operations, are no longer provided by some health authorities. Another method of explicit rationing relates to decisions made on the basis of probabilistic reasoning of treatments affecting a positive health outcome. One example was the case of 'Child B', who was unable to receive chemotherapy treatment for leukaemia on the grounds of the low probability of cure. Another is the denial of Coronary Artery Bypass grafts to people who smoke.

These forms of rationing have tended to encounter problems of public legitimacy as they involve potentially life-threatening conditions and have been associated with the suffering of particular individuals. There are also ethical objections to the criteria on which decisions about rationing are made, e.g. judgements about effectiveness or who 'deserves' health care. A number of these cases have met with adverse media coverage. The public toleration of such rationing strategies is likely to be limited, even though this sort of rationing has been operated covertly by medical practitioners for many years. Explicitness about the criteria used in making rationing decisions, it has been argued, is a more ethical way of rationing and prioritizing. Such an approach has been adopted by some UK health purchasing authorities during the 1990s (Øvretveit 1997). While this approach may appear to be more accountable, it does not guarantee public acceptability or escape the ethical dilemma that it relies on an approach which fails to respond to unmet need.

Waiting lists

Waiting lists incorporate both explicit and informal means of rationing. On the face of things waiting lists operate to manage demand according to rational criteria when demand outstrips immediate supply. In this sense they are seen to be operating according to equitable principles. The traditional assumption underlying waiting lists is that all referred patients have a valid potential need, which will eventually be met depending on resources, and patients with equal need will get treated on a first-come first-served basis. However, the waiting list system is not always an equitable way of dealing with demand because of the way it is managed. At the level of primary care more favourable waiting times for operations have been identified as a feature of fundholding practices (Audit Commission 1996). For some consultants it is a way of fostering demand for their individual practice by diverting demand from the NHS to the private sector. Patients with the ability to pay are able to reduce waiting times by seeing the consultant privately (Pope 1991). A supply problem may also be artificially created by restrictive practices, such as the non-maximization of operating theatre sessions by a proportion of consultants working in the NHS, which boosts demand for private treatment (Light 1997).

Co-payments

These are another means of managing demand, though they have not yet been used extensively in the NHS. They are likely, however, to be given further consideration as an available demand management strategy. In relation to social care, co-payments for home help and social care (e.g. payment for home help and long-term nursing care) have replaced services which were previously free. There are now muted suggestions of extending this to primary care, in the form of payments for GP visits and hotel charges for those admitted to hospital. Though co-payments have not traditionally been viewed as an overt means of rationing, they do have the effect of limiting demand: when the 1952 prescription charge was abolished by the Labour government in 1964 there was an increase in prescribing of 16 per cent (Allsop 1994). Other systems of care which have introduced co-payments for GPs, such as in New Zealand, have proved acceptable to population groups if the charges are not viewed as excessive (Croxyn, personal communication). However, introducing general practitioner fees has not, in itself, resulted in a decrease of utilization. For example, long waiting times have been found to have a greater impact on decreased utilization of services than fees (Gribben 1992; Cherkin *et al.* 1992).

Referral criteria, clinical guidelines and protocols

Medical decision-making guidelines and protocols based on valid evidence of best practice are aimed at the more effective management of health problems. Referral criteria are designed to ensure a reduction in use of unnecessary specialist hospital services. However, the costs involved in educating practitioners about these may militate against their being an effective demand management mechanism and the cost-effectiveness of this strategy awaits systematic evaluation (Øvretveit 1997). They may also be resisted because of their encroachment into the clinical autonomy of medical practitioners. At present, guidelines and information are geared towards clinical decision making and there are few examples of actively involving and disseminating guidelines to patients.

Modifying patient behaviour

Health promotion, promoting self-care and 'demarketing' have all been attempted as ways of modifying demand by modifying the public's behaviour. Specific behavioural interventions (discussed in Chapter 8) have also been designed for use in relation to specific groups of patients. Health promotion campaigns have to an extent been predicated on the assumption that encouraging healthier lifestyles can reduce the need for health care and have met with some success in reducing need which might otherwise have arisen (e.g. the Health of the Nation strategy; DoH 1992). More directly, self-care has been viewed as a means of promoting change in patient behaviour at the point when people become ill. The rationale is that encouraging the lay management of health reverses a passive reliance on formal health services. In the United States (US), demand management has been closely associated with giving people more access to information. The individual responsibility ethos running through this movement is indicated by this US employer's description of self-management strategies. Its aim is of 'softening the demand for services' in order to contain health care costs. It places the onus on employees to take more responsibility for people's health action:

> By offering employees the tools and know how to better care for themselves, the employer increases the likelihood that they'll use medical services more efficiently. No more trips to the emergency room for the sniffles, but also no more wait and see attitude when symptoms of potentially serious conditions, such as a heart attack, occur.
>
> (Ferkenhoff 1995)

In Britain, too, the use of self-care literature is beginning to form an important part of thinking about how to stem the tide of the rise in

demand for services such as out-of-hours care. The role of information is discussed in more detail in Chapter 8.

'Demarketing' refers to attempts to dissuade customers of the
need to use services. Demarketing as a strategy has been most
widely used in the US, where the need to dampen down supply-
induced demand for care has been greater than in the UK.[7] At two
points in the history of the NHS there have been attempts at what
might be viewed as the marketing of services. Meeting need at the
point of demand was the most saliently marketed feature of the
principles of the NHS (Seedhouse 1994). This 'marketing strategy'
has been remarkably successful. (Witness the resilience, over 50
years, of British public opinion about any modification of its social-
ized system of health care.) A second phase of marketing was
evident in the introduction of internal market arrangements in the
early 1990s. This ushered in new statutory health authority
responsibilities for assessing need and may have produced new
expectations about what health care should deliver. The theory of
planned behaviour derived from organizational psychology is being
used to change patients' patterns of use of services, through increasing the strength of a positive belief or decreasing the strength of a
negative one about a particular service (Marks and Elliott 1997).

THE ROLE OF LAY PEOPLE IN THE
FORMULATION OF DEMAND AND USE OF
SERVICES

Managing demand 'upstream' has led to a consideration of involving lay people in the way in which services are used. However,
views of patient involvement underpinning demand management
strategies seem at times to be predicated on predetermined and
simplistic views about the relationship between patient attitude and
action. There has been little in-depth analysis of the role of lay
people in using contemporary services. This has been expressed
succinctly by Allsop and Mulcahy (1996):

> The existence of standards, guidelines, rights and regulations
> will be of little use unless the patient is sufficiently knowledge-
> able to invoke these mechanisms, exercise their voice and
> change service delivery as a consequence ... The ultimate
> form of regulation is the patient or carer exercising power
> through being able to question the way that doctors define the

problem and the factors which have led them to recommend a particular course of action.

(Allsop and Mulcahy 1996: 139)

Attempts to involve people in debates and decisions about rationing have tended to take a superficial view of the potential and actual role of the participation of people in health care. Citizens' juries, for example, are predicated on the view that 10–12 individuals can represent the views of the lay public. Moreover, little acknowledgement is given to the fact that individuals fulfil different roles in making decisions about health care. Lomas (1997) points to the complexity of roles that people are involved with in decisions about health care. These include their roles as taxpayers, (with views about the funding of the health service), as patients (with preferences about the diagnostic and therapeutic interventions), and as local citizens (with a view about the services their local health care purchasers and providers should have on offer). Lomas's depiction of consumer roles is in keeping with a rationalistic approach to governmental policy concerns with efficiency and effectiveness. Others such as Allsop and Mulcahy (1996) stress the need to incorporate the 'life worlds' of patients[8] in policy analysis and implementation. This view of patient actions and roles is more centred on moral and practical questions and the wishes of patients to be treated as subjects to be properly consulted.

Consumerism has brought with it a focus on user behaviour and choice about services. This has highlighted the importance of the availability of information in making choices about and using health services. But for our analytical purposes, this consumerist perspective needs to be widened to incorporate other traditions of patient involvement and to understand the everyday concerns and contexts of people's involvement in health and health care. A consumerist approach also tends to be biased towards those who may already benefit disproportionately in relation to their need for health care. As Plamping and Delamothe (1991: 204) comment: 'clearly stated individual rights might benefit the powerful and articulate, but they will not do much for those who lack the means to negotiate for their own health'. A focus on those who currently do not benefit as much as they should from health services proportionate to their needs is more pertinent to understanding access to services. It is also relevant to the ability of services to meet unmet need. Expressed need and health action is intrinsically bound up with the socio-structural environment within which need arises (Rogers *et al.* 1997a).

In addition to consuming health care, lay people, like professionals, are providers as well as recipients of care. They have experience of self-care and care for others and are regularly involved in providing advice about, and taking responsibility for, health and illness (Cornwell 1984; Stacey 1988). The data we report later in this book suggest that patients are not only aware of the rationale and discourse of cost containment of public policy makers but that they make their own rational appraisal of these issues. This appraisal has an impact not just on the perceptions of services but also on the way in which people think about and make use of services.

Thus, a starting point for analysing the factors shaping the relationship between demand for, and use of, primary care is that ordinary people's perceptions are important. They are not only a barometer of the appropriateness and effectiveness of services, they are also a unique source of knowledge about the reasons, methods and timing of service utilization.

SUMMARY

Several observations can be made about the way in which the relationship between need and demand and the management of demand has been approached. The different emphases of need and demand highlighted by the discussion illustrate, first, that definitions of need for health care are contested and they reflect underlying tensions about knowledge and power. Second, notions of, and the process of, needs assessment have been relatively divorced from a policy concern with demand and the management of demand. In particular, need as a multi-dimensional and complex phenomenon fails to form a central place in demand management strategies. Moreover, 'the ability to benefit from existing service provision' as a criterion for defining 'appropriate' demand fails to acknowledge alternative ways of meeting need outside existing service provision. In describing the variety of current approaches to the management of demand, it is clear that the preoccupation with rationing has prevented more wide-ranging approaches to emerge.

In the final section the relevance was highlighted of focusing on the action of ordinary people as providers of health care and users of services in understanding the relationship between need, demand and use of health care. Drawing out the main themes of this first chapter, the next chapter concentrates on how the issue of inappropriate demand has been configured within the specific context of primary care. Chapter 3 extends the analysis of understanding need and demand by examining the literature and models deployed to understand the use of health services.

NOTES

1 The definition of the latter has broadened significantly in the post-war era as a result of medicalization and sociological and philosophical critiques (Øvretveit 1997).
2 Though commentators on health need more generally are increasingly advocating the need for explicitness. For example, in an editorial on need, Culyer notes that if the concept of 'need' is to be of practical utility then the value content of the term needs to 'be upfront and easily interpretable' (Culyer 1995).
3 For example, a widely used standardized measure is the Short Form 36 questionnaire (SF 36) which is designed to measure symptoms in the context of self-reported condition and the use of health care services (Lyons *et al.* 1994).
4 Equity, for example, is reduced to a problem of differences in rates of use of services between groups (Smaje and Le Grand 1997).
5 Just because there is no effective means of dealing with a problem does not mean there is no need. In its narrowest sense it also precludes the possibility of the development of effective or different ways of managing health problems. Aspects of quality of life and the multi-dimensional and relative notions of need are also important.
6 Evidence for the rise in demand for primary care is described briefly in Chapter 2.
7 In the US rates of inappropriate use of technology and the promotion of health care as a commodity means that the demand for health care has been stimulated more than in Britain where resources have always been rationed and the development and use of new technologies less widely available than in the States.
8 Lomas, for example, suggests that in involving lay people policy makers are looking to share some of the pain of rationing with the public (Lomas 1997).

2

THE PROBLEM OF INAPPROPRIATE DEMAND: THE VIEW FROM PRIMARY CARE

Society becomes more wholesome, more serene, and spiritually healthier, if it knows that its citizens have at the back of their consciousness, the knowledge that not only themselves, but all their fellows, have access, when ill, to the best medical skills that can be provided.

(Aneurin Bevan, *In Place of Fear*)

... I mean let's be honest about this, this has got damn all to do with improving patient care. That's a spin off, but the main reason it's done is because GPs are fed up with their on-call ...We should be honest with our patients and we should say, 'Look, we're knackered from this on-call; we hate it; we want to change it so that our lives are happier and, by the way, we'll try to maintain services such that you don't suffer', but it should be that way round.

(GP commenting on the introduction of out-of-hours co-operatives)

In this chapter we provide a picture of rates of primary care consultation and examine the way in which the issue of demand, particularly that considered inappropriate, has been formulated in primary care. Within the latter, demand has been defined mainly from the perspective of GPs judging the behaviour of patients in accessing services. However, organizational arrangements and professional behaviour are also important in driving up demand and this is also explored. As a corrective to the dominance of a service perspective on demands made by patients on primary care, towards the end of the chapter we will examine what a patient perspective contributes to our understanding of inappropriate demand.

PATTERNS OF CONSULTATIONS FOR PRIMARY CARE SERVICES

Differences in consultation rates have generally been explained by reference to three factors: *supply* factors (e.g. differences between the consulting hours and services offered by GP practices); *access* factors (e.g. distance from the practice) and *need* factors (e.g. mortality risk measured by ward standard mortality rates, chronic disease, life events, smoking and economic position).[1] The literature on the rates and reasons for differences in primary care consultation which are routinely collected as part of national and other surveys are generally divorced from discussions in the primary care literature about what does and does not constitute an appropriate referral. However, these are important in providing a backdrop to our subsequent discussion about meeting demand in primary care. There are several sources of data on the utilization of primary care services, in particular on the use of general practice services. The available data highlight the substantial use made of general practice services by the population and provide useful information on how the use of these services varies according to a variety of demographic and socio-economic characteristics (see Box 2.1).

Estimates suggest that about 78 per cent of those registered with a GP consult at least once a year. The most common reasons for consultation are respiratory conditions (31 per cent), diseases of the nervous system and sense organs (17 per cent), musculoskeletal disorders (15 per cent) and diseases of the skin (15 per cent) (McCormick *et al.* 1995). According to the General Household Survey (GHS) the average number of consultations per person per year is five (Rowlands *et al.* 1997).

The highest consultation rates are found among young children aged 0–4 and the elderly aged 75 and over (see Figure 2.1). For example, the average consultation rate for children aged 0–4 is seven per year compared with only three consultations for those aged 5–15. Overall women are more likely to consult than men. This is particularly true for the age group 16–44 years. Among this age group, the average consultation rate for women is six consultations per year compared with only three for men (Rowlands *et al.* 1997). Women are far more likely than men to consult their GP for genito-urinary conditions and diseases of the blood and blood-forming organs (McCormick *et al.* 1995).

Looking at marital status, there is little difference in consulting

---

**Box 2.1 Socio-economic characteristics associated with
increased likelihood of consulting: people aged 16–64 years**

Living in North or Midlands and Wales
Living in urban areas
Council property tenants
In other rented accommodation
Widowed and divorced
Living alone
Adults with young children
Social classes IV and V
Construction, service and industrial occupations
Long-term sick
Ethnic minority group
Smokers

Source: McCormick *et al.* (1995).

---

rates between those who are single and those who are married or
cohabiting. However, widowed and divorced people living without
a partner are more likely to consult than those who are single or
married (McCormick *et al.* 1995).

Consultation rates also vary according to household composition. Among men aged 16–64, those living alone have higher
consultation rates than those who are not. Both men and women
living alone are far more likely to consult for mental disorders than
those who live with someone else. Adults with young children in the
household are also more likely to consult than those without
(McCormick *et al.* 1995). There is evidence to suggest that the utilization of health services is associated with disadvantaged circumstances. For example, a higher proportion of people in social classes
IV and V consult in a year than those in social classes I and II.
Unemployment and being permanently sick are also associated
with higher consultation rates. Among men aged 16–44, those who
are unemployed consult their GP for mental disorders twice as
often as those who are employed. Consultation rates for serious illness are raised in all age groups for those living in rented accommodation, especially for respiratory and mental disorders. However,

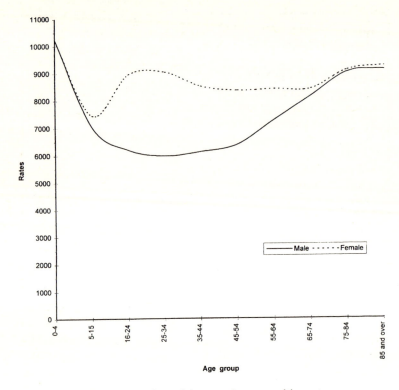

Figure 2.1 All diseases and conditions: patient consulting rates
Source: Derived from McCormick *et al.* (1995).

consultation rates for preventive health care are lower among those renting than among owner-occupiers. (McCormick *et al.* 1995).

There are relatively little data available on the use of primary care services by people who classify themselves as belonging to an ethnic minority group. Nevertheless, the research data that are available point to differences in consultation rates between different ethnic groups. The Health Education Authority commissioned a series of health and lifestyle surveys, of which two surveys were specifically targeted at ethnic minority groups. These surveys found evidence of higher GP consultation rates among African-Caribbeans and South Asians than among the general population. For example, it was estimated that the average number of GP consultations per person per year is 4.2 among African-Caribbeans, 5.0 among Indians, 7.1 among Pakistanis and 7.9 among Bangladeshis, compared with only

3.6 for the whole UK population (Rudat 1994). A recent analysis of General Household Survey (GHS) data suggests that while there does not appear to be any gross inequity in the use of general practitioner services between ethnic groups, the Chinese population have consistently low levels of use. There is also some suggestion of underuse of services by women of Pakistani origin. Additionally, low referral rates of ethnic minority groups to outpatient departments might be an indication of inequitable referral between primary and secondary care (Smaje and Le Grand 1997).

There is some indication that high need for primary care services is localized. Adults aged 16–64 living in urban areas are more likely to consult their GP for any reason than their counterparts living in rural areas. However, similar differences are not found among children and the elderly. Profiles of the relationship between health need and consultation have suggested greater comparative disadvantage and associated use of services in practices situated in the most deprived areas (Hopton and Dlugolecka 1995). Looking at regional variations in consultation rates, men aged 16–64 living in the North of England, the Midlands or Wales have higher consultation rates than those living in the South of England (McCormick *et al.* 1995).

All these studies focus on GP consultation and offer little insight into patterns of consultation for other services within the formal primary care sector or health care which is managed outside formal services through, for example, alternative therapies, self-care or informal care from other lay people. Chapter 7 focuses on pharmacy consultations, while consultations with, and use of, alternative practitioners are briefly explored next.

Alternative practitioners

The use of alternative therapies has not, until recently, been viewed as a legitimate focus for understanding patients' help seeking behaviour. As Sharma has commented: 'most of the studies which have used the concept of lay referral have tacitly assumed that the main choices open to the patient consist of consultation with a medical doctor, self treatment or no action at all' (1990: 31). The extent of use of alternative therapies raises the question of the extent to which popular consumer-based demand in an increasingly market-orientated society can diminish established patterns of provision (Saks 1992). Less is known about the use of alternative therapies than general practice and pharmacy.

With regard to the extent of use, there are no large cross-sectional data available on alternative practitioner utilization and few British surveys provide us with accurate estimates of the extent of utilization, need and demand. However, the available data do suggest that use is increasing over time. In Wadsworth *et al.*'s 'clinical iceberg' study (1971), carried out at the beginning of the 1970s, less than 1 per cent of people sought help from lay healers. Both the availability of, and demand for, alternative therapies have increased in recent years and more contemporary studies suggest a far higher rate of referral. Estimates of the number of people who have consulted complementary therapists at some time vary from one-fifth to around one-third of the population (Furnham 1994). Consultations with alternative practitioners represent between 6.5 and 8.6 per cent of the number of consultations with GPs each year – between 11.7 and 15.4 million consultations per year (Fulder and Munro 1985). However, many of these consultations are for ongoing treatment of a chronic problem. Primary care consultations representing the first point of call in an illness episode are likely to be far less.[2]

Data from community studies (e.g. Furnham and Forey 1994) suggest gender differences in levels of use of alternative therapies, with between 27–29 per cent of men compared with 33 per cent of women making use of such treatments. There is also evidence for variation by age, with a substantial proportion in some age groups (60 per cent at age 35 and 80 per cent at 45 years) reporting having tried alternative treatment at some time. Little is known about the choices made by different ethnic groups in relation to alternative medicines, or about regional differences within the UK. Despite the gradual changes that have been seen in recent years in the scale of use, demand for alternative therapies is likely to be related to restricted access, with ability to pay or registration with a fund-holding practice determining access.[3] Figures suggest that the expenditure in this sector is considerable. As we will examine in more depth in Chapter 8, the culture of alternative therapies has also permitted changes at the level of self-care. Annual sales records from one leading manufacturer, for example, reported that sales at retail were worth £18 million in the last financial year. With estimated growth in the purchase of remedies directly by the public being in the region of 15–20 per cent per annum for the last five years.

The data presented above provide a picture of the pattern of use of primary care. Additionally, Accident and Emergency (A and E) services are frequently used as a form of primary care. This is discussed in more detail below. We now turn to the position and role that general practice has had in the overall policy of meeting demand within the health service.

GENERAL PRACTICE AND MEETING DEMAND

A founding tenet of the NHS was access to care free at the time of need. General practice was that part of the health service structure considered to be best placed to fulfil this principle. Since the inception of the NHS, the GP has provided both the initial generalist medical response to health problems and, in assessing the needs of the individual, has acted as a gatekeeper to a range of other health service and social resources. However, the status ascribed to general practice in managing the bulk of health problems at the interface between local communities and the NHS has not until recently been reflected in the status that it has been ascribed. Rather than being seen as the epicentre of the health service, until very recently it has been politically dominated and overshadowed by secondary and tertiary care sectors.

The policy priority in the 1990s of a 'primary care-led' NHS was a strategic attempt to re-establish primary care as the pivotal point of service provision. Concern about rising demand has been a feature of the rationale for this change. Providing more care at the interface between the community and general practice might reduce the need for more expensive secondary care intervention because as a gatekeeper to secondary services, primary care has the potential to keep supply costs down. Actual or perceived rising demand and the need for cost containment have increased interest in the savings which might accrue from the use of less expensive primary care staff. In this regard the view has been expressed that primary care-led purchasing is likely to result in better and more cost-effective treatments for patients (Roland and Wilkin 1996).[4]

In addition to the expectation that primary care might increasingly contain and manage demand for the NHS as a whole, there has also been an interest in levels of demand at the interface between the public and general practice. Overall, primary care consultations do not appear to have risen markedly in recent years. Nor, with the exception of discharged long-term patients of psychiatric hospitals, does existing evidence show that a shift in services from secondary to primary care has resulted in increased workload for GPs (Pedersen and Leese 1997). However, these broad indications of relative stability in demand levels over time mask some specific changes. There has been a significant rise in demand for out-of-hours services (Hallam and Cragg 1994), and some practices have recorded very large increases in the number of consultations for specific population groups or conditions. For example, one practice recorded a rise in the average number of consultations for children in each of the first years of life (discounting developmental surveillance and immunizations) from 3.73 per child in 1960 to 17.2 in 1990 (Del Mar 1996). As discussed in Chapter 1, the cause or causes of such rising demand for primary care are not clear. They are likely to be a combination of patient demand and/or changes in remuneration and practices on the part of primary care professionals. Increases in GPs' fees and the hours at which they could be claimed, introduced in 1990, proved an incentive to increase the number of visits GPs' undertook. In 1967 four out of hours fee claims per 1,000 visits between midnight and 7.00 a.m. were recorded. In 1993, with a more generous time coverage of 10.00 p.m. to 8.00 a.m., fee claims reached 35 per 1,000 visits (Hallam 1994). Additionally, alongside a marked increase in demand for out-of-hours visits is evidence that, for the vast majority of GPs, time spent 'on call' has decreased with the introduction of larger practice rotas (Electoral Reform Ballot Services 1992).

What is clear is that the out-of-hours commitment has become a vehicle for expressions of professional dissatisfaction. At the same time it has had the effect of concentrating attention on the problem of managing and reducing patient demand. Discontent among GPs with the principle of 24-hour responsibility for patients became a focus of dispute between them and the Department of Health when negotiating their new contract in 1990. Increased daytime responsibilities (such as health promotion), at a time when there was a need for cost-containment strategies, led to medical pleas to reduce night-time commitments to patients. The negotiated contract reinforced the GPs' right to choose whether and where a consultation takes place and was thus designed specifically to circumvent the need to visit patients in their homes outside normal surgery hours (Electoral Reform Ballot Services 1992; Hallam and Henthorne 1998). A singular analytical and empirical focus on *patient* factors tends to obscure or marginalize these professional and policy influences on the conceptualization and construction of the 'problem' of rising demand.

THE CONSTRUCTION OF THE PROBLEM OF INAPPROPRIATE DEMAND IN PRIMARY CARE

Policy documents have emphasized a 'clinical' perspective on meeting need in primary care. At the same time they stress the requirement for primary care to be able to respond to the 'vague' and 'undifferentiated problems' presented by patients (DoH 1996). In the main, the construction of inappropriate use of services emerges from GP judgements about patient behaviour. The focus on inappropriate demand within primary care seems to centre on the very services which patients have considerable discretion and freedom in accessing. Hence there has been a particular concern with the use of A and E and out-of-hours services. Patients themselves initiate these types of service contact and the professional must respond to uncertainty set by, or imposed by, the client, not *vice versa*. The literature relevant to inappropriate demand extends to:

* types of consulting patient,
* consequences for the practitioner of dealing with inappropriate consulters,
* imputed causes and solutions to the problem.

Studies of general practice carried out in the 1960s and 1970s conceptualized the problem of inappropriateness as the presentation of 'trivial' problems. More recent analyses have added to this formulation by incorporating the phenomenon of the 'heartsink' or 'difficult' patient (Ellis and McGuire 1986; Gerrard and Riddell 1988; O'Dowd 1988; Dowrick 1992). Ideal types of 'good' and 'bad' primary care patients were presented in the work of Stimson and Webb's (1975) study of GP views. 'Good' patients were deemed by GPs to be those who fit in with the way in which GPs prefer to treat patients. This included a preference for male and middle-class patients with clearly defined diagnosable problems, where the patient was amenable to action by the GP. More recently, the concept of 'heartsink' appears to have intuitive appeal among GPs:

> . . . there are patients in every practice who give the doctor and staff a feeling of 'heartsink' every time they consult. They evoke an overwhelming mixture of exasperation, defeat and sometimes plain dislike, that causes the heart to sink when they consult.
>
> (O'Dowd 1988)

Similarly 'frequent attender' is a term applied to the 'minority' of patients who consult frequently and are considered to have a 'disproportionate' effect on clinical workload and present multiple problems to GPs (Neal *et al.* 1998). Consultations by certain kinds of patient are considered more appropriate than others. These include those who are anxious, elderly or very young; those who have mobility problems; or those who would suffer severe distress from not visiting the doctor (Lattymer *et al.* 1995). By implication those who do not fit into these categories are considered to be inappropriate consulters. Categories of difficult patients (Gerrard and Riddell 1988) include those who repeatedly consult but do not get better; those who are culturally very different from the doctor and those whose consultations stem from family rather than individual problems.

A recent study (Lattymer *et al.* 1995) on out-of-hours services found that key elements of GPs' attributions of appropriateness included the degree to which patients were viewed as assuming responsibility for and participating in:

* self- and mutual treatment for the condition,
* a willingness to travel to see the doctor, and
* an acceptance of telephone advice.

Those identified as having 'social problems', making calls for non-clinical reasons or 'misunderstanding' the purpose of the out-of-hours service were considered to form inappropriate demand.

Studies of inappropriate use within primary care tend to be biased in favour of the subjective feelings evoked in GPs by patients. For example, in one study (O'Dowd 1988) the use of the concept of 'heartsink patient' is justified on the grounds that:

> . . . while it lacks the charm of many neologisms, it is nonetheless descriptive. Ellis's term 'dysphoria' is more elegant but sanitizes a messy feeling and focuses attention away from the sufferer onto the patient. 'Heartsink' more clearly refers to the doctor's emotions which are triggered by certain patients.

Patient blaming is inherent to these definitions and discussions of 'heartsink'. Little room is made for alternative explanations which extend beyond the patient's behaviour, knowledge or attitude or a purported breakdown in 'communication' between GP and patient. This patient-defect model is in marked contrast to other espoused primary care traditions towards consultations, such as the 'biopsychosocial' model (Dowrick *et al.* 1996). Holistic models recognize that psychosocial factors and context are legitimate parts of patient care in consultations.

The construction of the problem of inappropriate consultation may also be linked to the status of general practice as a profession. It has had difficulty asserting itself as legitimate and equal to other medical specialties. As was pointed out earlier, for some time after the setting up of the NHS, GPs operated in the shadows of their hospital counterparts and so the profession attempted to emulate hospital medical practice. Dealing with minor trivial and uncertain problems fits uneasily with this aspiration, as pointed out by Calnan and Gabe (1991):

> the recurrent concern about trivial demands, the desire for hospital work, and the emphasis on academically acceptable foundations are all examples of the continuing influence exerted by the consultants over their generalist colleagues.
>
> (Calnan and Gabe 1991: 145)

The concept of the 'difficult' patient might also point to professional difficulties when diagnosing or managing uncertain conditions such as psychosomatic disorders. Recent research suggests that general practitioners are as uncertain as their patients in knowing what to do about certain symptoms (e.g. chronic fatigue syndrome) (Fitzgibbon *et al.* 1997). Seen from this perspective, 'heartsink' patients may signify a projection of doctors' own difficulties in coming up with an appropriate response in terms of diagnoses and management. A label of 'heartsink' may provide a convenient evasion for the GP – 'if in doubt blame the patient'.

ORGANIZATIONAL AND PROFESSIONAL FACTORS SHAPING DEMAND

In considering how demand is generated, the dominance of the 'patient blaming' discourse described above obscures the role of the GP and primary care organization. Yet a number of studies suggest that a significant amount of demand is generated by doctors themselves, with estimates varying from one-third to three-quarters of all consultations (Morrell *et al.* 1971) concluded in their study on the rates of consultation that: 'the biggest single factor affecting the proportion of return consultations, and therefore workload, is the doctor himself'. In a study of one practice by Armstrong *et al.* (1990), the need for reattendance was judged to be nearly three-quarters of the patients who had attended for an initial consultation. This study also found that the control of doctor-initiated consultations was limited not only by clinical considerations but by the difficulty doctors had in accurately communicating advice on reattendance to patients. In terms of the relevance of poor communication for determining future demand, Armstrong and colleagues concluded:

> In principle clear guidance to patients on whether to re-attend should help to control workload because, on the one hand, a rational plan of re-attendance for those who need it may deter causal consultations or minimize the risk of future problems, and, on the other hand, clear advice to those who do not need to re-attend may prevent inappropriate consultations in the future.
>
> (Armstrong *et al.* 1990: 242)

In addition to these practitioner factors, which induce reattendance, there have been rapidly changing aspects of service delivery, workforce and commissioning arrangements. Changes in service delivery and professional behaviour are likely to have redefined the parameters of services in responding to, and shaping, need and demand.

Changes in professional roles and perspectives

One change includes the theory underpinning training, practice and involvement in aspects of care previously dealt with by the secondary care sector. Changing GPs' working arrangements and their training may also act to widen the areas of need which primary care workers consider to be within their remit, which in turn may increase patient demand. For example, new models are being developed which underpin GPs' responses to health care problems better suited to everyday medical problem solving. Professional leaders have for some time promoted GPs as 'primary care specialists' and 'family counsellors' and these conceptions are evident in the policy statements of the Royal College of General Practitioners (RCGP). One of these recent statements extends the remit of the GP to spiritual and holistic elements of care (RCGP 1995). The inclusion of 'new' health and social problems or the introduction of 'needs' previously dealt with in different ways can also be expected to generate 'new' demands from patients. For example, routine testing and counselling for HIV within primary care is relatively new (Van Castern *et al.* 1993). Also GPs are being urged to become involved in the identification and treatment of new problems, even where such a need has not been formulated by the patient. For example, the notion of the somatization of psychological symptoms derives in the main from liaison psychiatry, and perceived need for treatment for psychogenic conditions may be lower among patients than GPs (Veerhaak and Tijhuis 1992; Karlsson *et al.* 1995). Changes in skill mix within the primary care workforce are also likely to influence patient demand. In particular, the introduction of nurse practitioners as a means of GP substitution may impact on the nature and degree of patient demand by discouraging some demand or encouraging the duplication of consultations if their role is less acceptable to patients in dealing with certain illnesses.

Organizational and service arrangements in primary care

There is some evidence that characteristics of general practice are influential in shaping patient demand. Patients of single-handed practices, for example, have been shown to consult more frequently for ongoing and minor illness and be more likely to have contacted the practice out of normal working hours than patients of group practices (Hopton and Dlugolecka 1995). Single-handed practices are also less likely to be running health promotion clinics than group practices (Gillam 1990) so demand for such services is likely to be less in patients registered with single-handed practices. Changes in the appointment systems for primary care medical and nursing consultations can change patterns of demand. It is interesting to note that GPs in the USA reduced their workload by offering same-day appointments for all consultations. After the introduction of this system consultations fell by 8.3 per cent a year (*Pulse* 1998). In the UK the introduction of a telephone triage for managing acute illness in general practice during the data resulted in a fall in doctor workload by 54 per cent over a three-month perod (Gallagher *et al.* 1998).

A failure on the part of primary care to deal quickly and responsively with expressed need which is most appropriately dealt with by the secondary sector may result in a continuing burden of care at the primary care level. For example, it has been shown that the most deprived groups in the population are more likely to consult a general practitioner with symptoms related to common conditions of inguinal hernia, gallstones, tonsillitis, varicose veins, cataract and osteo-arthritis but were generally least likely to receive surgery (Ben-Shlomo and Chaturvedi 1995).

Organizational arrangements and service response in Accident and Emergency departments

An inter-relationship between primary care and A and E services exists in relation to levels of demand. First, the public have considerable discretion in directly accessing this service instead of, or in addition to, primary care services. Second, at an organizational level inappropriate demand for A and E services is frequently seen as *appropriate* demand for primary care services. Increases in attendances at A and E departments have been attributed to a number of factors (e.g. morbidity and social deprivation). Research suggests that people identified as using A and E services 'inappropriately' may prefer these to GP services for a number of reasons, including:

- the anticipation of long delays in seeing the GP and of subsequent referral from the GP. For example, Calnan (1983) suggests that lay people may discriminate about which source of help to access on the basis of their complaint: visiting A and E if their problem needed technical experience, such as dressing a wound, and visiting the GP if they needed to discuss symptoms,
- patients' failure to understand the organizationally designated role of the A and E department (Green and Dale 1992),
- satisfaction with GP is associated with low attendance at A and E (Hallam 1994),
- access and proximity have been associated with the propensity to use A and E services (Green and Dale 1992),
- responsiveness of service compared to primary care out-of-hours. Hallam (1994) found that 3–6 per cent of patients have attempted to contact a GP before visiting the A and E department (Hallam 1994).

That patient demand is in part determined by the nature of the A and E service provided rather than being predominantly a characteristic of patients is encapsulated in the following comment in a nursing article on the subject: 'if the professional view of what is appropriate cannot be enforced, perhaps the label "inappropriate" belongs to the A and E services rather than the patient' (Walsh 1995).

Organizational and service arrangements in other parts of the NHS and beyond

It is likely that changes in the provision of services outside and at different points in the NHS will influence demand for primary care services. Statutory changes in other parts of the welfare sector may also have an impact on primary care demand. For example, the recent Childrens' Act focuses attention on meeting the assessed needs of children with disabilities and requires the involvement of both general practitioners and community child health doctors in identifying and assessing need (Bhrolchain *et al.* 1993). The level of provision of educational psychology by local authorities affects the level of demand for primary care consultations about a range of emotional difficulties in children (Finney *et al.* 1991). Problems previously seen by local authority child care services may, as a result of reductions in these services, place new pressures on primary care. There are similar changes in relation to assessment, surveillance and care arrangements between local authorities and other agencies in primary care, in community care in general and community mental health care in particular. GPs, including fundholders, are expected to be involved in developing and contributing to care management programmes alongside other health and social services (Audit Commission 1994).

Providing services differently at the primary and secondary care interface, such as the relocation of outpatient clinics from the secondary to the primary care sector, may also impact on the levels of activity within primary care. Patients previously accessing the secondary sector may now be more likely to turn to GPs for care following such changes (Macdonald and Macdonald 1992).

New computerized monitoring and record-keeping systems

New computerized monitoring and record-keeping systems may have a more general impact on patients' demand. New management systems have been set up in many practices. These systems have been found to enhance the utilization of services, e.g. in the reduction of dropouts from the immunization programme (Singh *et al.* 1992). Calling back patients for routine checks and reassessment of medication may be a source of new demands. This process is illustrated by the following account from a woman in our 'Pathways to Care' study (PTC) who would not have attended the GP surgery unless she was 'sent for':

> *I have to come periodically to have my blood pressure checked, every three months. I should come to him for that; I don't always remember, but I do come, I mean, I do have to see him because if I don't come it's on the computer and they, in fact they send for me. He [the GP] said to me: 'Mrs K it's over six months since I've seen you.' I said: 'Is it really?' . . . Well I suppose it's because it's all computerized now – they know quicker, don't they?*

Indirectly, organizational arrangements and professional conjectures are incorporated into patients' assumptions about when it is appropriate to access care. Cartwright (1979) identifies three reasons why patients may consult their GPs for minor ailments which are likely still to be relevant to contemporary primary care use:

- The service may be viewed as trivial and therefore appropriate for minor illness.
- The lack of definition of the scope or range of primary care services can lead to it being seen as appropriate for minor illness.
- The inaccessibility of other sources of professional help may encourage people to present their needs in terms of illness. Other professionals may be seen as more appropriate but primary care is the only place to which people have access.

With regard to the first of these, a number of aspects of primary care service are identified which suggest why patients may legitimately view primary care as the appropriate place for dealing with minor ailments. These include:

- the length of consultations (often less than five minutes),
- the place of consultation; hospitals are seen to deal with major health problems and events (such as birth and death) and in comparison primary care is viewed as the place to consult for mundane routine problems,
- the nature of the help given, particularly the infrequency of

physical examinations conducted by GPs, and the use of prescribing as a means of trivializing the consultation or making
things easier for the doctor,
- awareness that general practice does not have the specialist
  equipment to deal with problems other than trivial ones,
- the fact that patients are encouraged during the consultations to
  present and discuss a single complaint which may trivialize a
  more complex problem.

CONVERGENCE AND DIVERGENCE IN PATIENT AND MEDICAL PERSPECTIVES ON APPROPRIATENESS OF DEMAND

Studies of GP views about the appropriateness of the use of services rarely consider the perspective of patients. More patient-ori-
ented research suggests that there is a concern among most people
not to 'bother' professionals without good reason, and a desire not
to be perceived to be consulting unnecessarily (Eyles and Donovan 1990; Irvine and Cunningham-Burley 1991; Punamaki and
Kokko 1995a). There is some evidence too that patients' notions of
appropriateness are negotiated during the process of help-seeking
and doctor and patient interaction. A study by Punamaki and
Kokko (1995a) found that prospective patients had an 'internal'
dialogue, which could include a defence of their reasons for consulting and an assessment of the lay and professional responsibilities in diagnosing and treating illnesses. Additionally,
patient-assessed successful consultations were dependent not on
doctors and patients starting with similar interpretations of illness,
as previous empirical work had suggested, but on an interactive
process of negotiating the cause of symptoms and treatment. The
character and content of the patients' explanations for their complaints were important predictors of whether the consultation was
perceived to be successful. Patients who had either a biomedical or
experiential model of illness were less likely to be unhappy with
the consultation than patients who had an eclectic explanation
which subsumed both physical and subjective elements. Patient-
assessed predictors of successful consultations included doctor
friendliness towards the patient, and the professional volunteering
of information and explanations. In particular, patients valued

their feelings and perceptions of illness being taken into account as an integral part of the consultation (Punamaki and Kokko 1995b).

Roberts (1992), in a review of the use of health services, using the search terms 'misuse', 'abuse' and 'inappropriate', notes a tendency of both medical and social science literature to conceptualize the patient as a passive recipient rather than active participants in care. According to Roberts the medical literature viewed parents presenting ailments of their children as being irresponsible or misguided. Social scientists have acted as apologists or advocates for patients, explaining inappropriate attendance in terms of poor access to GPs, mistaken beliefs about the relative skills of hospital doctors and GPs, and lay health beliefs. In a subsequent study of minor ailments presented in A and E, decisions to seek help were not found to be irrational (as perceived by health care workers). They were based on a rational appraisal of the situation in which it was difficult to predict the outcome of illness. It also included a need to act responsibly as a parent. Assessments were also made on the basis of what might happen rather than on an evaluation of existing behaviour.

The issue of inappropriate demand is likely to be linked to different notions of self-limiting illness held by professionals and patients. This is illustrated with reference to a study of a common complaint presented in primary care, urethral syndrome, viewed from a medical perspective as being a self-limiting illness. From a lay perspective, the persistent and frequently recurring pattern of symptoms makes it a more long-term problem that is viewed as requiring medical intervention (Pill 1987). Pill notes the tactics used by GPs to tackle such problems, such as closing down rather than opening up the consultation. This may increase the GP's sense of control but may not be conducive to promoting self-help, as this GP's comment illustrates:

> Opening up the consultation implies losing control – what if this patient poses problems to which there is no answer? What if the patient expects this kind of consolation every time she comes? Will I make her happier anyway? Will I end up with a lot of this kind of patient dependent on me?
>
> (Pill 1987: 282)

In the face of evidence of incongruence between doctors' and patients' perceptions of the nature and severity of problems, the most prominent policy/practice responses have focused on the need for improvements in 'communication' and in doctor–patient relationships. Differences between doctor-defined and patients' self-assessed needs have also been judged to be exacerbated by differences in social background; specific knowledge and experiences of ill-health; and ability to control the utilization of medical care between the patient and the medical practitioner (e.g. Magi and Allander 1981). Dowrick (1992) suggests there is a need to explore the possibility of a lack of congruence between doctor and patient in much greater depth. He also theorizes that the 'heartsink' referral is a failure in communication which can be resolved by locating health and illness behaviour in the context of a person's background and general beliefs. In his case study of problematic consulting behaviour of one family, he explores the tensions that exist within a particular practice, such as retirement and 'quick staff turnover' and argues, *contra* Balint (1956), that far from mirroring the patient's feelings in an attempt to facilitate understanding, the doctor's own tensions and experiences can get in the way and preclude such comprehension.

Part of the professional discourse on inappropriateness describes the negative impact on the individual medical practitioner's well-being and on his or her competence as a practitioner. An unsuccessful consultation, for example, is one which is portrayed as being distressing for both doctor and patient (O'Dowd 1988; Dowrick 1992). Negative effects on the GP include reduced confidence in dealing with patients, or in clinical ability, and unsuccessful interactions with patients are a common source of occupational stress (Winefield and Murrell 1992). The effects on practice are argued to include the possibility of missed diagnoses or inferior treatment because of the poor quality consultations which are perceived to flow from lowered self-confidence and professional self-image (Dowrick 1992).

Some of the concerns about the consequences of 'inappropriate' demand, highlighted in the literature on GP perspectives, mirror concerns about unsatisfactory consultations with GPs from the patient's perspective. Irvine and Cunningham-Burley (1991), for example, suggest that mothers' unsatisfactory consultations on behalf of their children can result in loss of self-esteem and trust in the doctor–patient relationship, making future decision making about health more difficult. Similarly, mutual understanding, good communication, and the need for each other's perspective on health and illness to be valued, are seen to be prerequisites for positive consultation. This suggests that there may be a significant degree of consensus between lay people and doctors about the factors that are important, not only in the doctor–patient relationship, but in what comes to be defined as 'appropriate' use of services. However, the potential to exploit this consensus is masked at times by the assumed lack of validity of a patient perspective. In one study GP respondents expressed the view that public involvement in the debate about proposed changes in out-of-hours care would, through increased awareness of the presence of the service, lead to greater use of primary care services (Lattymer *et al.* 1995). This suggests a lack of professional trust among some GPs in patients' ability to be discriminating and rational in their decision making about primary care service utilization.

The area of most tension between primary care doctors and the public is in the use of out-of-hours services. People are increasingly being given messages that they must not call out the doctor 'inappropriately' and are being made to feel increasingly guilty about the use of such services. At the same time doctors are seeking ways of reducing their commitment to providing out-of-hours care as a way of reducing their overall workload in the context of their concerns about rising commitments and the length of their working day. This is illustrated in recent press coverage (see Boxes 2.2 and 2.3).

Seen from the GPs' perspective, patients often consult out of hours with symptoms which they have been experiencing for several days. It is felt that a high proportion of calls are unnecessary or could have waited until the next day. Patients are seen to be consulting with symptoms similar to those presented daily in GPs' surgeries, with only a small minority having had no opportunity to have arranged a consultation during normal surgery hours. According to this GP perception, only a small proportion would have suffered harm had they waited for a normal opportunity to consult (Hallam and Henthorne 1998). However, what seems to be lacking from this interpretation is an analysis of the process of help seeking and an understanding of the motives and context of patient decisions to access care outside normal hours. Such views do not consider the limitations of the symptom-based model with which to make judgements about the appropriateness of consultations more generally (discussed in more detail in the next chapter).

Moreover, research suggests that most decisions to make use of out-of-hours services are not generally taken in a cavalier manner and that there is an awareness that it is a limited right to be able to call on the doctor's time. Decisions appear to be made against the

Box 2.2 Bedside manner fails to impress doctors on call

They do not feature in any medical text book, but every GP is familiar with them: the bizarre calls made in the small hours of the morning by patients who view their family doctor like the local pizza delivery man.

Despite efforts by medical organisations to deter trivial calls, patients persist in phoning their GP for advice ranging from the mundane to the highly personal, according to a survey.

One 82-year-old woman called up Dr Thomas Abraham of Hull at dawn one morning complaining she had been awake since 4.30am seized with 'an irresistible desire for sex'. Wisely refusing to leave the security of his own bed, Dr Abraham offered her advice over the phone. He declined to visit 'for reasons of personal safety.'

Dr Timothy Woodman, from Gillingham, Kent, was called by a woman at 3am who wanted him to remove her sleeping daughter's contact lenses. He, too, declined to leave his bed.

A Birmingham GP told of being called on a Sunday evening for help with a crossword on the grounds that the answer was a 'medical word', and another in Grays Thurrock, Essex, declined to visit a patient complaining of 'excess wind'.

The survey, by the medical magazine *Pulse*, also records the case of a woman who walked from her home in Hornchurch, Essex, to her GP's surgery – only to ask for a home visit as her phone was broken.

A British Medical Association spokeswoman said out-of-hours calls to GPs had risen fivefold over the past 20 years.

Source: Article by Jeremy Laurance, Health Editor in *The Independent*, 13 May 1997, reproduced with permission.

backdrop of the unacceptability of calling out of hours and with the acknowledgement of the exceptional circumstances and the unacceptability of calling the GP out for minor things (Hallam and Henthorne 1998).

Box 2.3   Anger over ban by doctors

Family told by practice that their first call-out in 25 years was a 'gross abuse of the system'

A Cheshire GPs' practice yesterday came under fire for striking off a family who called out an emergency doctor for their sick daughter – their first call-out in 25 years.

Michael and Janice O'Grady were told by Stephen Maxwell, a partner at the Kenmore medical centre in Wilmslow, that they had wasted resources and abused the system by calling out an emergency doctor when they feared that their eight-year-old daughter, Sara, had contracted meningitis.

The family has now had to register with another doctor. They have lodged a complaint with the local health authority, and next week will embark on the formal procedure aimed at resolving the dispute.

Mr O'Grady, a 50-year-old retired headmaster, said yesterday: 'We find it totally abhorrent that our first emergency call, when our daughter was extremely distressed, results in us being removed from the list.'

He said his wife, a medical secretary, had obtained a price list for emergency locum services that suggested the call-out may have cost the practice as little as £12. 'I have offered to pay that. At the time, I would have paid £100 to get a doctor to see Sara.'

The practice's decision was yesterday described by the Patients' Association as 'outrageous'.

Martin Bell, the local MP, also voiced concern. 'I haven't heard the doctor's side,' he said. 'But if it is as Mr O'Grady says, then it does seem an extraordinary case.'

Media inquiries to the practice were yesterday being referred to the Medical Defence Union. A spokeswoman said Dr Maxwell was not prepared to comment because doing so would breach patient confidentiality.

The dispute began on December 8 when Sara was sent home from school complaining of nausea and a headache. During the afternoon, she also developed a temperature so her parents called the practice and were told to take Sara to the emergency surgery.

When they arrived to be told that they faced a 90-minute wait, they informed the receptionist that they would return in an hour. But as soon as they got home, Sara vomited, then fell asleep. Her parents decided to leave her in the hope that she would sleep off whatever she had been suffering from.

But when she awoke a few hours later, her condition appeared to have deteriorated. 'She was screaming for something to take away the pain in her head,' said Mr O'Grady. 'We just panicked and called the doctor.'

An emergency locum attended and prescribed antibiotics for an infection – but only after Mr O'Grady received a phone call from Dr Maxwell, in which, he claims, the GP accused him of 'not being bothered' to wait at the practice.

On Christmas Eve, the family received a letter from Dr Maxwell, informing them that the call-out had been an 'expensive waste of resources' and a 'gross abuse of the system' and that they had been removed from the list.

Although the individual GP with whom they were registered, David Stockley, has accepted Mr and Mrs O'Grady's version of events, the practice has refused to reconsider. 'All I want is an apology,' Mr O'Grady said yesterday.

Source: Article in the *Guardian*, 27 January 1998, reproduced with permission.

SUMMARY

This chapter has focused on understanding perspectives about appropriate and inappropriate demand for primary care services. The issue of appropriateness of use is bound up with the expanding remit of primary care services. In attempting to place boundaries around their work, GPs have focused on inappropriate demand, particularly in relation to out-of-hours commitment as a vehicle for expressions of professional dissatisfaction. The perspective from primary care professionals is on inappropriate patient behaviour. It tends to ignore other possible explanations and perspectives. This provides a skewed focus on the use of services by the patient in a way that does not fit primary care provider norms. Organizational arrangements and professional behaviour are at least equally, if not more, implicated in generating demand. Other literature suggests there are a complex set of factors influencing the patient's decision to use primary care. Decisions to contact out-of-hours services are made against a backdrop of awareness about limited resources, of GP reactions and of expectations of patients to ration the use of services. The current literature on GP and patient perspectives remains unsatisfactory unless it is linked with an analysis of help seeking and health care utilization. The next chapter provides that link.

NOTES

1 This approach is critically examined in the next chapter in the context of critically scrutinizing models of health utilization.
2 There appears to be no survey estimating the use of alternative practitioners defined in this way. However, from a qualitative study examining the use of alternative therapists, only 20 per cent of the sample used therapists as a first port of call in an episode of illness (Sharma 1990).
3 A recent national survey shows that fundholding practices are significantly more likely to offer complementary therapies to their patients than non-fundholding practices.
4 Although doubt has been shed on the ability of GPs to act as purchasers for whole populations.

MODELS, APPROACHES AND PROBLEMS IN THE STUDY OF THE USE OF SERVICES

It is obviously easier to study or to treat the individual and even easier to blame the individual for health problems or failures to seek medical care promptly, than to consider problems of health in a more inclusive framework.

(A. Alonzo, *Social Science and Medicine*)

INTRODUCTION

In the last two chapters need and demand were examined in the context of contemporary health services and primary care policy. In this chapter, the focus shifts to a description and assessment of the frameworks commonly used to understand help seeking and health services utilization. Of all the models evaluated, we conclude that the social process approach appears to be the most promising for examining help-seeking behaviour. It is this latter approach which is adopted in subsequent chapters.

In comparison to the US, there has been little British development of health utilization models and concepts. This is because until recently NHS care has been assumed to be universally and easily accessible to most of the population, most of the time. The highlighting of a lack of access to services for some population groups, (e.g. ethnic minorities), the introduction of overt 'rationing' and cost-containment strategies, together with a recognition of the impact of personal financial resources on the problems experienced by certain population groups which may affect their use of services, radically undermine this assumption.

The study of the use of services has been viewed as following the contours of the major contributing disciplines within Health Services Research (HSR). In making sense of aspects of health policy, social scientists have made reference to different traditions analysing problems, e.g. the economic, sociological, epidemiological and public health perspectives. Similarly, in his review of studies on utilization behaviour, McKinlay (1972) outlined a number of ideal types of research. These included:

- *The economic approach* – focuses on the factors relevant to transforming need into demand. These include: income, health insurance cover, the cost of health services and the availability of free medical care.
- *The geographical approach* – focuses on the proximity and locality of services as a determinant of utilization behaviour.
- *The socio-demographic approach* – identifies the patterning of service use according to variables such as age, gender, social class, education, etc.
- *The socio-psychological approach* – refers to work which has approached utilization behaviour with reference to motivation, perception and learning.
- *The socio-cultural approach* – has directed attention at the study of values, norms, beliefs, definitions of situations, and life styles associated with utilization behaviour.
- *The organizational approach* – refers to the impact of organizational phenomena on utilization behaviour, in particular the assumptions and response of those working in organizations to people using services.

Like all 'ideal types' these approaches were not intended to be viewed as mutually exclusive and certain types of factors in help-seeking behaviour can be found in each of the models. McKinlay's typology is important for two reasons. As a result of inter- and multidisciplinary working within health services research, there has been a substantial integration of different aspects of each of these approaches (Pescosolido and Boyer 1996). Both the health belief model (HBM) and social behavioural model have integrated to an extent the interests of other disciplines. Also, the 'clinical iceberg' model is claimed by both epidemiology and medical sociology. None the less, the emphasis on some factors more than others suggests different understandings of need, demand and use, which are still represented by differing disciplinary perspectives. Thus, in this chapter we are concerned with critically examining five approaches to understanding primary care and health service utilization. These are the 'clinical iceberg' studies which, from an epidemiological perspective, examine the patterning of service use according to rates and type of symptoms in the community. The social-psychologically orientated HBM includes psychological and social characteristics to predict individual help-seeking behaviour. The rational choice and economic models of decision making are influenced by economics and view decisions to seek help as a rational weighing-up of costs and benefits by individual social actors. The fourth approach we discuss is the social behavioural model which has situated individual characteristics within the context of the organizational and other socio-political aspects of health care systems. Finally, the social process approach to entry into health care focuses on decision-making processes and lay action in accessing care and is considered the most appropriate model for assessing the use of services in a way which helps us understand the social situations and contexts underlying people's illness behaviour in using primary care services.

CLINICAL ICEBERGS, SYMPTOMS AND CONSULTING RATES

The literature on the 'clinical iceberg' (non-referred symptoms) reveals that individuals are rarely asymptomatic. Past studies of symptoms, whether involving self-reports of illness or other epidemiological measures, suggest that most symptomatology does not come to the attention of the health services. Unreported health problems have been conceptualized in the medical literature as 'a clinical iceberg' which is sometimes also referred to as a 'service gap', between need and utilization of services (Cleary 1989). Kookier (1995) suggests that the nature of the iceberg differs in emphasis according to disciplinary or professional foci. Whereas epidemiologists and some social scientists are concerned with the 'iceberg of morbidity', because of an interest in gaining accurate estimates of the amount and distribution of disease in the population, medical practitioners are interested in the 'clinical iceberg' – serious undetected symptoms related to diseases such as glaucoma, diabetes, tuberculosis – which require the attention of clinicians. Thus the two definitions of icebergs overlap but are not identical.

A number of studies have sought to estimate the proportion of symptoms that result in consultation within primary care and/or to explore the type of symptoms involved in consultation compared with non-consultation. Though the popularity of undertaking these studies was at its height in the 1960s and 1970s, more recent studies show similar results in terms of the existence of a large number of 'unreported' symptoms. In the 1960s, Wadsworth and his colleagues (1971) found that 95 per cent of their sample had experienced health complaints in the two weeks preceding the interview, but only 20 per cent had sought medical help of some sort, with the largest proportion, (12 per cent) visiting a family doctor. Research also suggests that the ratio of unreported to consulted symptoms varies according to the type of symptom experienced. Using a health diary in which patients recorded their symptoms daily over a one-month period, Banks *et al.* (1975) found only one episode in 184 headaches was presented to primary care services compared to one in 18 sore throats. In another study, Scambler *et al.* (1981) interviewed 74 working-class women and found that only one in 74 subjects who suffered 'nervous depression' or irritability consulted her GP, compared to one in nine for sore throats. There is also evidence that consultation is positively linked to severity of symptoms. There is little in the way of a clinical iceberg for life-threatening conditions and evidence that unreported symptoms are milder than reported ones (Ingham and Miller 1982; Verbrugge 1984; Waldron 1983). However, there is greater complexity when specific sets of symptoms are examined. For example, there is some evidence to suggest that a proportion of people who are suffering from extreme pain do not seek help. Hannay's study of 1344 patients registered with a Glasgow health centre also suggests that while they may be less severe, symptoms not reported to primary care are not necessarily trivial. This study assessed the prevalence of subjectively defined symptoms and referrals in terms of pain, disability and perceived seriousness (Hannay, 1979). He estimated that what he referred to as 'the medical-symptom iceberg' (where symptoms were assessed by the respondent as severe but did not result in consultation) was two and a half times the size of possible 'trivia'. Similarly, a survey of the health status of a sample of individuals who underwent extensive medical tests found that 57 per cent of those in the sample who had previously not visited their GP with a complaint were subsequently referred to their GP (Kookier 1995). More than a fifth of the symptoms made known to GPs for the first time were considered serious enough to warrant referral to hospital or specialist services. Other studies have shown that while the majority of unreported health problems may be mainly minor illnesses such as headaches and fatigue, there is also some evidence to suggest that more serious symptoms remain unreported (Huygen *et al*. 1983; Kookier 1993; Stoller and Kart 1995).

Co-morbidity and types of symptom also complicate matters and have necessitated the development of more sophisticated models with which to understand the relationship between symptoms and health services utilization. The presence of psychiatric morbidity has been associated with an increased consultation rate for physical problems (Magi and Allander 1981) and patients with significant symptoms of depression have been found to have higher rates of health services use more generally than those without (Callahan *et al*. 1994). Barsky *et al*. (1986) developed a five-stage model of utilization corresponding to the configuration of somatic and psychological symptoms. Physical symptoms were conceptualized as:

> a final common pathway through which emotional dysphoria, psychiatric disorder and socio-environmental stress as well as organic disease are expressed . . . In addition hypochondriacal attitudes, specifically disease fear and bodily preoccupation, appear to be significant factors in medical utilization.
>
> (Barsky *et al*. 1986: 559)

Notwithstanding the increasing sophistication of attempts to explain health service use with reference to symptoms as the main drivers, there are limitations to this approach for understanding the relationship between need, demand and use of services.

The limits of morbidity as an explanation of help seeking

The focus on symptoms as the main explanatory factor in consulting behaviour has a number of limitations. There are disagreements, both among professionals and between professional and lay people, over the notions of the existence and interpretation of symptoms. Existing methodologies are inadequate for clarifying whether differences lie in bodily sensations or in the social and psychological meaning and experience attached to these. Bodily feelings, including symptoms, are given meaning by being compared with previously stored experiences (Skelton and Pennebaker 1982). This was evident in the research conducted by Punamaki and Kokko (1995b) on patient decision making in seeking primary care discussed in the last chapter. Rather than focusing on the meaning of morbidity, others have preferred to pay more attention to the situation within which it arises and to view 'illness behaviour' as arising from an interaction of biophysical feeling, social and psychological interpretation and evaluation. In this regard, inter- and intra-psychic processes are important in the containment and management of physical symptoms. Mechanic (1961), for example, has argued that symptom reporting reflects a pattern of illness behaviour that is influenced largely by the affective state of the individual and that utilization models based on symptoms fail to account adequately for the psychosocial triggers of help seeking (Mechanic 1979).[1]

Counter-intuitive patterns of health service utilization also suggest there are limitations of symptoms as indicators of health need and use. As we have discussed above, at times the duration of symptoms is negatively related to the use of medical care and those with severe symptoms do not necessarily consult more (Berkanovic and Telesky 1981; Meininger 1986; Briscoe 1987). Similarly there are consultation variations in different population groups despite the presence of similar morbidity. Rather than long-term disability placing ever-increasing demands on services over time, demands for health care may at times decrease over time. Experienced patients may resort to personal coping strategies or alternative sources of help with the progression of their illness careers (Brown *et al.* 1994; Borkan *et al.* 1995; Bendelow 1996). Bendelow's qualitative study of the careers of patients with chronic pain showed that some patients accommodated to their symptoms by the self-management of pain. Patient strategies, reinforced by lower expectations of services through contact over time, played a more important role in the management of symptoms than accessing and using formal health care services.

Symptom-based studies are also limited in explaining primary care utilization for the large number of consultations concerned with uncertain, chronic and 'illegitimate' complaints. The latter have uncertain aetiology and pathogenesis and include repetitive strain injury, hypoglycaemia, candidiasis, multiple chemical sensitivity, myalgic encephalomyelitis and chronic fatigue syndrome (Adamson 1997; Cooper 1997). Managing these conditions implicates existential uncertainties for patients and clinical uncertainty for professionals treating them. The traditional view has been the undesirability of the medicalization of some of these problems from the patient's point of view and the wish to find certainty among medical practitioners. In a reversal of other means of managing clinical uncertainty, where it has been assumed that the nature and course of a disease will be overcome by the eventual discovery of new medical findings, procedures, experiments, and standards of rationality, it is lay organizations which are pushing for a more medicalized approach to uncertain illness. Primary care physicians and others, in contrast, are arguing for the need to demedicalize conditions such as myalgic encephalomyelitis (ME). Sufferers of ME are more likely to diagnose their condition than their doctors, and often come to the consultation equipped with extensive knowledge (Scott *et al.* 1995).[2] In the next section we consider psychological studies of illness behaviour and how they might help us to understand the gap between symptoms and the use of services.

THE HEALTH BELIEF MODEL AND OTHER PSYCHOLOGICAL EXPLANATIONS

Developed over the course of the last three decades, the health belief model (HBM), and the rational choice and socio-behavioural models, together form the three dominant theories of health care utilization. Health psychology has tended to examine factors such as traits, attributes, personality and attitudes in the seeking of care. It argues that people perceive symptoms differently and accordingly will act differently. A prominent model is the social psychologically-orientated health belief model (HBM). First developed to explain preventative health behaviour (Kasl and Cobb 1966), it has also been adapted to explain illness behaviour and help seeking. The HBM uses a cognitive framework which emphasizes 'vulnerability' and 'barriers' to help seeking and includes psychological and social variables with which to predict individual behaviour. According to this model: 'readiness to seek medical care is determined by perceived benefits and barriers to seeking care and cues that instigate appropriate behaviour' (Rosenstock 1966: 53). This model has been developed to take account of four sets of variables attributable to individual help seeking, which are then correlated with whether or not help is sought. These four sets of variables are:

- readiness to take a particular course of action,
- perceived risks and benefits from uptake of health care,

- internal and external cues to action (e.g. internal cues like pain or external ones such as interference with everyday life),
- modifying factors (e.g. gender, age, ethnicity, class, personality).

Analytical models developed from this approach have been applied to the use of specialist services for specific conditions.[3] A number of studies have suggested that high users of services perceive themselves to be ill and vulnerable to illness (Ingham and Miller 1982; Blaxter 1985; Murray and Williams 1986; Cook *et al.* 1990; Mackay 1990). Low users of primary care, on the other hand, express less anxiety about illness, are less concerned about symptoms, are more likely to be critical of doctors, and less convinced of the efficacy and benefits of medical treatments (Egan and Beaton 1987). High users are those who fit more into the ideal type of compliant patient and adopt a more passive 'doctor knows best' attitude. Locus of control and coping are also concepts aligned with the HBM approach. 'Locus of control' (LOC) relates to the degree of personal control a person considers he or she has over the cause and course of illness and its outcome. External locus of control refers to the location of threats to health emanating from outside an individual's control, whereas those who are in possession of internal locus of control are construed as believing that they have a high degree of personal control over their health. External control has been identified in those who are 'high' users of general practice services, internal control being associated with low use of primary care (Ingham and Miller 1982). In relation to uptake of primary care preventative screening and checks, internal LOC appears to be positively related to 'self-screening' activities such as breast examination over which there is a high degree of personal control whereas external LOC is positively related to physician-dependent screening activities such as cervical smears (Courtenay *et al.* 1974). The fact that those who are high users of primary care and those who are more likely to use medically dependent health promotion screening are also more likely to adopt a 'doctor knows best' attitude and to perceive themselves as having lower personal control over their health. This questions the assumption that health promotion in primary care is able to promote self-care and health-enhancing behaviours in a way which will act to decrease primary care demand for illness.

Formal help seeking has been seen as one of a number of coping mechanisms deployed by lay people in dealing with stress

(Gourash 1978). The concept of coping from a psychological perspective usually refers to the adaptiveness of a person to a particular situation and the ways in which people react to life stress through particular cognitive–behavioural, avoidance or situational strategies. Health care utilization can be viewed as a response to a problem when other informal support strategies fail (e.g. keeping busy and ignoring or denying the problem; Saunders 1993). There is a mixed picture regarding the extent to which coping style is related to the seeking of formal care. Vulnerable groups who have higher rates of illness but low ability to cope have been found to make greater use of services than other population groups (Barker *et al.* 1990; Blount *et al.* 1992; Attias *et al.* 1995). For example, it has been found that people with problems of anxiety who use cognitive avoidance and rumination reduced the propensity to seek help from services (Vollrath *et al.* 1993). However, studies suggest that coping style and resources are not directly related to service use. Repression or sensitization to illness has been found to be associated with differences in the reporting of symptoms and response to common symptoms but not related to frequency of visits (Antonovsky *et al.* 1989; Barker *et al.* 1990). There is also some evidence that one coping mechanism – for instance, the accessing of formal health care – does not substitute for another.

Finally, other psychological explanations outside the HBM are also notable in the literature. There is also a small body of literature which has examined lay attributions of illnesses which are viewed indirectly as linked to consulting behaviour. For example, using a structured questionnaire, Furnham (1994) examined lay people's beliefs about the importance of overcoming five illnesses commonly referred to primary care. The most important factors were found to be inner control and understanding the availability of help on offer to deal with the illness.

The psychological literature on illness behaviour extends our understanding beyond the notion of symptoms as an explanation for help seeking from formal services, to an understanding of relevant psychological contingencies. Patient preferences have been of particular importance in understanding patient decisions to use services. Moreover, over time the HBM has broadened its focus to include factors considered central in other approaches. The earlier models focused mainly on individual factors to the exclusion of other social and systemic influences. The revised versions have been more inclusive. For example, within the framework of 'reasoned action', social networks are considered as important in reinforcing 'normative beliefs' about service use.

Limitations of the psychological model

The assumptions underlying traditional psychological approaches do not always accurately reflect the action of people, tend to ignore the role of meaning and context in the purposeful action of individuals, and downplay the importance of social networks and other social processes. In relation to the first point, one criticism of the notion of 'readiness to act' centres on the failure of a health belief model to predict behaviour accurately, since the accuracy of the model can only be judged *post hoc* (Dingwall 1976). A psychological model assumes that a relationship exists between individual traits (in the absence of patient accounts) reflected in health beliefs and rates of service use. Within this model the patient is seen as being open to external influences or 'cues to action', for example, advice from others, previous episodes of illness and media reporting. However, not only are 'cues to action' difficult to measure in cross-sectional research but the behavioural focus of psychological approaches also tends to view these 'cues' without reference to the meaning attributed to these by individuals or the context and extra-individual factors which may account for attitudes and action. For example, the concept of locus of control is applied to the attitudes and behaviours of individuals with little attention paid to social context except as an extraneous variable. It has been suggested that the measures of multidimensional locus of control fail to illuminate the relationship between social–structural position and control over health-related behaviour and that a more fruitful avenue of research would be to examine the relationship between beliefs about control over more important aspects of an individual's life such as work (Calnan 1983).[4] The same lack of attention to the autonomy of individuals and their social context in decision making is apparent in the literature exploring the role of health professionals in developing coping strategies among patients and carers, where professionals are given the role of 'guiding' lay people into positive ways of acting and 'coping'. What is missing from this professional discourse is the way in which lay people themselves define coping and useful coping strategies, how these might inhibit or promote formal health service demand and use, and how professionally perceived notions of positive coping strategies might map onto these.

A further weakness in psychological models relates to the importance attributed to individual behaviour at the expense of other variables (Bloor 1995). A growing body of qualitative research, exploring different aspects of people's perceptions of fate and control, highlights the significance of social processes which are related to the individual's perception of the cause of ill health. Thus, notions of 'fatalism' have been found to be strongly related to realism in the lives of people (Blaxter and Paterson 1982; Pill and Stott 1985; Davison *et al.* 1991; Howlett *et al.* 1991). It has been suggested, for example, that the 'fatalistic' attitudes towards health and illness identified in black and Asian groups may be attributable to the effect of racism and racial oppression in and outside the health service (Howlett *et al.* 1991).

Finally, the HBM in particular and psychological research in general underplays the potential that lay or 'common sense' knowledge has in understanding utilization behaviour. Instead, priority is given to psychological interpretations and terms such as 'cognitive avoidance and rumination', 'ineffective and maladaptive ways of dealing with stress', or 'dysfunctional family systems'. Little consideration is given to whether lay people themselves view their behaviour as 'maladaptive'. Indeed, the notion of health belief rather than knowledge contains the a priori assumption that lay views are inferior and may be invalid. In contrast to this approach, research which takes seriously people's own accounts of health behaviours viewed as negative from an official point of view (e.g. smoking) suggests that substantial benefits can be derived from adopting health-denying behaviours (Graham 1987). Overall, much psychological work currently fails to view help seeking as a process involving the action of a number of people, action which takes place within a social context which influences behaviour to a much larger extent than individual psychological traits.

RATIONAL CHOICE MODELS OF DECISION MAKING

The 'rational choice' model of decision making is prominent in the health economics literature and health care decision-making research more generally. From this perspective, lay decisions are viewed as 'purposive' and as being made by individual social actors who weigh up the costs and benefits of a particular action in situations with variable characteristics, constraints and opportunities. The model assumes that in making a decision, people begin by determining whether he or she stands to lose or win according to some reference point. The individual who, having preferences and being confronted with constraints, has to make choices. The individual within this model is viewed as an egotistic, rational utility-maximizer.

The rational choice model has been adapted in the health care literature by dropping what are considered to be unrealistic non-economic phenomena. Its main advantage for work on lay decision making about help seeking is that it fits the increasingly consumerist philosophy of health care and the assumptions of people more generally in advanced capitalist societies (Pescosolido 1992). The rational choice model of decision making has been used most extensively in examining decisions made by health care professionals and, to a lesser extent, patients' decisions about specialist interventions. These include decisions to undergo amniocentesis, the termination of pregnancy or other forms of surgery (Kahneman and Tversky 1979, 1984; Marteau 1989). These are procedures which can be framed most easily as having certain risks and benefits, (e.g. invasive procedure versus amelioration of symptoms) and therefore fit the model best. This approach is less powerful for, and more infrequently used in, understanding decisions made by lay people in open systems (as in primary care). The emphasis on health care interventions rather than processes of entry into health care relates to an assumption that demand for care and help seeking is only relevant in terms of the value of the outcome of the care itself:

> Patients seek care in order to be relieved of some actual or perceived present or potential, 'dis-ease'. The care itself is not of direct value; it is generally inconvenient, often painful or frightening . . .
>
> (Evans 1990: 118–19)

The assumption that there are no gains for patients in the seeking of care is a questionable one. The advantages of the process of seeking care are recognized by GPs. They are known, for example, to place patients on a waiting list as a means of reassuring patients that they will be seen some time in the future. The advantages for patients in help seeking are discussed in detail in Chapter 5.

One attempt to develop a model of demand for medical care which takes account of lay decision making to undertake self-care and seek formal primary health care is the episodic approach to the demand for health services. This views decision making as a continuum which ranges from no action to a decision to seek health care. Thus it is inclusive of decisions which lead to 'self-care' that may not lead to utilization. This model provides a corrective to traditional utilization measures which prioritize volume of users and numbers of physician visits and is a better reflection of medical care (Bentzen *et al.* 1989). Applying this model in a Danish diary study examining patient choice and use of primary and self-care, the authors found that symptoms of longer duration were those where people chose to use the doctor, and that self-care was used in relation to symptoms of shorter duration.

The emphasis on decision making within the rational choice approach has the advantage of recognizing the role of patients' action in influencing demand. However, the extent to which help seeking or entry into health care is a matter of rational *decision making* is a moot point. The notion of decision making as a concept relevant to help seeking and use of services is rarely questioned. The type of decision being made in the health arena is different from decisions made in a different context. The decision to seek help is a 'depth' as opposed to a 'casual' decision. 'Depth decisions' are those which have important consequences for the individual and are composed of a number of stages whereas casual decisions (e.g. the choosing of a consumer durable) are much simpler and have less significant implications and consequences for the individual (Kadushin 1966). In relation to the use of private medical care, Calnan and Cant (1992) found evidence that decisions were influenced by resource issues, particularly regarding concerns about time, finance and subscriptions (i.e. the benefits of circumventing waiting lists balanced against the risks of increased premium payments). They noted, however, the passivity of the patient in challenging the GP as the gatekeeper to the private sector and found little evidence of the systematic weighing-up of costs and benefits. Additionally, rather than a protracted conscious assessment of options, decision making around minor disorders rotates around a three-stage 'brief and straightforward' process involving the identification that something was wrong, assessment of significance and a decision to act.

Active decisions about health are not always made. In an illness situation it is a truism to point to the fact that a series of decisions can be made. Whether they are made is another matter. As Selznick pointed out some time ago: ' "Decision making" is one of those fashionable phrases that may well assume more than it illuminates.' It certainly does have an 'air of significance of reference to important events', and the mere use of the phrase does seem to suggest that 'something definite has been scientifically isolated' (Selznick 1957). The overturning of decisions and non-action is also important to consider, as well as 'abortive illness' behaviour, in which 'contingencies' and 'new topical relevances' intervene in a way which promotes or inhibits help seeking. For example, in a study of illness behaviour among residents of a lodging house, Bloor (1985) found that people sought to guard their work routines against disruptions by illness and that the demands of the work situation led people to accommodate illness rather than seek immediate help.

The concept of 'choice' as a motivator to action and the attribution of rationality as an inherent feature of decision making also downplays habitual behaviour as the basis of health action. This is illustrated by an extract from Robinson's study of help seeking for primary care among a sample of families living in Wales:

> From the analysis of the South Wales data it became apparent that a series of clear-cut overt decisions . . . was rare. Neither were there many long drawn-out series of assessments . . . For the most part the principal actors in any illness situation did not consider more than one course of action. There was no thinking out and weighing up of alternative strategies to obtain a series of defined goals, when, for example, mothers put antiseptic cream on grazed knees, took aspirin for a headache, kept children in the house when they had chills, or called in the doctors when someone's temperature was found to be 102. These mothers knew what to do and did it . . . in what sense is this behaviour rational?
>
> (Robinson 1971: 35–6)

Choice is only one way of entering health care. For example 'coercion' and 'muddling through' are relevant constructs with which to understand help seeking in relation to particular health care services (Pescosolido *et al.* 1998). Additionally, in real-life situations lay evaluations of costs and benefits may take a different form and a range of factors that may not be included in the traditional rational choice model may be important. In our pathways study of help seeking, there were indications that people self-rationed their seeking of care, and that this was influenced by an awareness of a resource-constrained NHS and the cost of services.

SOCIO-BEHAVIOURAL APPROACH TO UTILIZATION

The socio-behavioural approach has been developed to explore the factors that shape different types of general medical health care utilization in different contexts (Andersen 1968; Kroeger 1983). In relation to medical consultation for minor physical and psychological problems, for instance, Anderson and Newman (1973) have used path analysis within a behavioural model in an attempt to understand differential levels of access among sub-groups of the US population. The socio-behavioural models rest on three sets of factors which constitute the basis of an individual and rational decision-making process:

1 *Enabling factors* – relate to the accessibility of resources (financial and geographic). The concern here is with issues of access to care and the organizational characteristics of the health system. Enabling characteristics reflect the available means, knowledge and ability to act which are needed to use health care. These include geographical availability; having a consistent and regular source of care; travel time; and financial ability which limits or promotes the use of services.
2 *Need variables* – relate to the nature of the illness. This refers to aspects such as severity and type. The nature of illness refers to both biophysical aspects of illness and social and psychological aspects such as the hurt, worry or bother a condition may cause.
3 *Predisposing factors* – these concern the predisposition to use services suggested by demographic social characteristics and beliefs about services.

In Anderson's study of an American non-institutionalized population between 1975 and 1976, the direct effects of illness were found to be the main determinants of physician visits. A similar linear, structural equation model was used to study the effect of these variables on physician utilization in Norway (Arne *et al.*

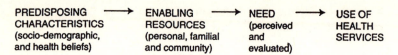

Figure 3.1 Socio-behavioural model
Source: Anderson (1995).

1983). This analysis found that illness and need variables, as measured by number of disability days and psychological well-being, were 'almost exclusively' the only important variables in explaining health service utilization. In relation to three enabling factors – travelling time, work hours and number of children (a measure of family obligation) – only the last of these was found to be important in explaining service use. Over time Anderson revised the socio-behavioural model by incorporating more variables measuring the organizational structures, goals and policies of different health care systems (Anderson 1995).

There are a number of limitations to the socio-behavioural model as used in these and similar studies. While there is acknowledgement in theory of social, environmental, and provider factors which might affect consultation – socio-demographic characteristics, perception of illness, whom one consults – these are underdeveloped in empirical work (Phillips *et al.* 1998). As heuristic devices, these models have been found wanting. For example, they are limited in explaining delays in the seeking of care and reasons underlying patterns of referrals (Anderson and Newman 1973; Eraker *et al.* 1984). This may be because rates of illness at each point in the model appear to be the basis of assessing need, which suggests that symptomatology is still the primary focus for the analysis. Second, the model works on the basis of a clear distinction between the provider and recipient of care. The influence of people outside the formal sector, or the possibility that people will manage illness in ways other than consultation with a doctor, are not considered. Third, the focus is still on the outcome, not the process or interactive features of decision making. Fourth, the model is best for accounting for acute conditions requiring hospitalization; it is less relevant for accounting for illness trajectories and use of care for more chronic groups, and for the fact that much more formal care (e.g. primary health and social care is community orientated).

HELP SEEKING AND HEALTH CARE USE AS
SOCIAL PROCESS

The American sociologist Elliot Freidson noted that a drawback to the type of models just discussed were that they tended: 'to emphasise choice over constraint, the individual over the group, the actor over the environment' (1970: 63). Similarly, in an early review of research into help seeking, McKinlay (1972) notes a general tendency for researchers to concentrate on the *decision* to seek care rather than the *decision-making* process. Research on the process of decision making from within medical sociology and social psychology since then has tended to move away from motivation and determinants of decision making as fixed attributes of individuals. The social process approach to utilization focuses on the *interaction* of the patient with others, and views motivation and determinants of decision making as subject to the influence of a wide range of factors often beyond an individual's control. Central to this conceptualization of help seeking is the notion of illness as a social rather than a medical category.

Social process approaches to health care utilization have drawn heavily on the notion of illness as a social entity and the concept of illness behaviour. Illness behaviour has been defined by Mechanic as 'the manner in which persons monitoring their bodies define and interpret their symptoms, take remedial action and utilise the health care system' (1980: 1). From a functionalist perspectives Parsons (1951) argued that illness was the inability to fulfil one's role, while Freidson (1960) suggested that the criteria by which lay people judge illness are related to norms about bodily experiences or normal capacity. Parsons's work on the sick role included a focus on the obligations and responsibilities which set the parameters for people to seek help and enter the sick role and patient role. Other social scientists have since placed greater consideration on how individuals define and cope with illness as an everyday experience (e.g. Fitzpatrick *et al.* 1986). They have viewed the defining of illness as a selective, interpretive and evaluative process taking place within a specific social context, and have drawn attention to the ability of people to use a combination of health care advisers and means of dealing with illness simultaneously.

The illness career approach, rooted in the symbolic interactionist and labelling or social reaction perspective within sociology, drew attention to the way in which the patient role is negotiated and maintained, and how others react to and categorize illness. Stages in the illness career have been described as a combination of a set of changes to self identity; stages in a medical condition; psychological and personal response to social environment; and contact with institutions and their personnel (Clausen and Yarrow 1955; Goffman 1961; Roth 1963). The illness career approach has similarities to the socio-behavioural model in that it conceptualizes a set of phases which people embark on in a progressive and directional manner. It differs in so far as the experience of illness is viewed as a set of logical critical decision points which are flexible and where 'alternative decisions at any step can lead to further decisions or to a reconsideration of earlier ones' (Twaddle and Hessler 1977: 155).

During the 1960s and 1970s a number of social models of pathways to care were suggested for understanding help-seeking behaviour. Mechanic (1961), for example, identified three stages of the help-seeking process: the illness stage during which the problem exists and is recognized; the illness behaviour stage during which attributions for the problem's existence are made and various coping strategies are attempted; and the help-seeking stage during which the individual seeks professional help. He argued that these stages were also influenced by symptom-related factors, including the frequency with which the illness occurs in a given population; the relative familiarity with the symptoms of the average member of the group; the relative predictability of the outcome of the illness; and the amount of threat and loss which is likely to result from the illness. The first two dimensions refer to the problem of illness recognition and the latter two to the problem of illness danger. Mechanic also made a distinction between problem recognition and attribution as interrelated but separate processes and has provided evidence that these are learned responses and that individuals vary in their predilection to do either (Mechanic 1979, 1980). Zola and his colleagues (1973) examined the process of referral in a sample of people experiencing minor disorders and from this identified five non-physiological triggers to the referral process:

1 The occurrence of an interpersonal crisis.
2 Perceived interference with personal/social relations.
3 The 'sanctioning' of ill-health in one individual by another. (On occasions individuals sought the sanctioning of their ill-health and complained when it went unnoticed.)
4 Perceived interference with vocational/work-related activity.
5 Temporalizing of symptomology – 'if it doesn't get better by . . . I'll see a doctor'.

In a North American context Alonzo (1980) developed a process model based on a situational understanding of illness and the containment of symptoms which addressed the way in which acute illness came to be presented to formal services. Six analytic care-seeking phases were defined:

1 *Prodromal or warning phase:* the period between initial awareness of health deviation and the onset of acute symptoms.
2 *Self evaluation phase:* the period between acute symptom onset and the seeking of advice from lay or medical others.
3 *Lay-evaluation phase:* the period between seeking lay advice and the decision to seek medical evaluation.
4 *Medical evaluation phase:* the period between the decision to seek medical evaluation and the decision to travel to the hospital.
5 *Hospital travel phase:* the period between initiation of hospital travel and arrival at the hospital.
6 *Hospital evaluation phase:* the period between hospital arrival and arrival at an appropriate hospital bed.

In-depth qualitative research which used unstructured and semi-structured diaries of illness behaviour and decision making about illness was also undertaken in Britain (e.g. Robinson 1971; Dingwall 1977). Such work has provided a rich conceptual and theoretical basis for subsequent research on illness behaviour and lay knowledge in medical sociology, although it has not always informed policy making in the NHS as much as it perhaps could have done. Research which has been informed by a social process approach suggests that the following are important in relation to health, need, demand and use of contemporary primary care:

- the relevance of examining the timing between the onset of problems and consultation,
- the extent to which people are able to contain and cope with signs and symptoms within socially defined situations and contexts,
- the multiple possibilities in the decision-making process including the overturning of decisions and non-decision making as well as the reasons for seeking out formal help,
- the relationship between everyday events, activities, work and decisions to use primary care,
- social networks in decisions to seek help.

Each of these aspects is discussed further in Part II.

BRIDGING THE GAP BETWEEN MODELS OF USE

> Patterns of care describe the combination of advisors and/or
> practices that are used during the course of an illness episode.
> Pathways add the additional element of order, that is the
> sequences of advisors and/or practices used over the course of
> an illness episode.
> (Pescosolido and Boyer 1996, describing the network
> episode model)

Pescosolido (1991) draws on the 'illness as career' models by viewing
medical decision making as rooted in a process whereby decisions
made at any stage are shaped by those made at an earlier stage. Five
decisions are considered central to the process of coping with illness:

* recognition (the decision that something is working),
* utilization (the decision to seek care),
* initial compliance (the decision to follow medical advice),
* outcome (recovery, death, disability or chronicity),

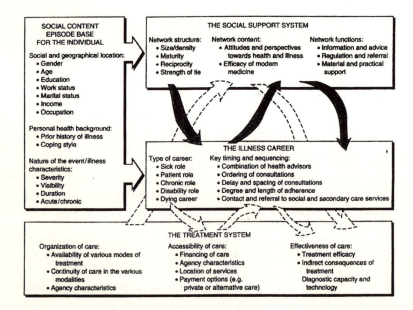

Figure 3.2 Network episode model (adapted)
Source: Pescosolido (1991).

- secondary compliance (the decision to continue in a long-term treatment regime).

The social organization strategy and the network episode models (Pescosolido 1991) seek to include the advantages but exclude the disadvantages of the rational choice approach to understanding decision making. They also implicitly incorporate elements of a social process and pathways to care model which allows for entry into the health care system to take a variety of forms. The focus is shifted, therefore, from choice by the individual to socially constructed patterns of consultation decisions. In so doing, this model acknowledges the importance of social characteristics in the differential use of services. Social interaction and social networks are incorporated into the mechanisms for seeking help, together with notions of purposive action, economic and psychological rationality, and 'utility maximization' drawn from the rational choice model of decision making. The focus of this approach is not only on who receives care but *when* and *how* care is received (Pescosolido and Boyer 1996). Central to this framework is the assumption of heterogeneity among groups of individuals who seek help from medical practitioners and the power of social networks to influence use which, like services, might also change over time. The testing of this approach using a secondary data set illuminated the complexity of decision making and the myriad possibilities involved in help seeking and pathways to care in an American context. (Data from our own research about patterns of help seeking and use of self-care are presented in Chapter 5.) Pescosolido and others point to the importance of common-sense knowledge derived from past experience and people's relationships with others outside the formal health care system. The latter can be 'short or momentary, planned or spontaneous, supportive or controversial'. The essence of this framework then appears to be the need to situate an understanding of the management of an illness in a context which incorporates elements of both formal and informal health and social resources, and to pay attention to the reserves and resources of living in communities which are relevant to consider during a course of illness. This is the focus of elaboration in the next three chapters.

SUMMARY

The approaches to health care utilization discussed above provide an extensive listing of contingencies that affect the use of services.

These contingencies range from the psychological in the HBM (for example, patient preferences) to the external environment in the socio-behavioural model (including policy context). A number of limitations have been discussed in relation to the frameworks described above. While they are of considerable use in providing a rich picture of the range of contingencies relevant to the use of formal services, they also have considerable limitations for developing a research agenda which aids our understanding about the help-seeking processes relevant to contemporary primary care.

Inherent to the three types of contingency models described in this chapter is an approach to an understanding of who seeks care and why, by focusing on correlates of decision making through quantitative surveys or indices (Pescosolido 1991). To a large extent traditional models share an underlying assumption of consistency in individual preferences, perfect knowledge and the ability and wishes of individuals to make probability calculations in a similar way to experts. While it is likely that these are features of patient decision making, it is unlikely that they are the only ones, or perhaps even the most important factors explaining the way in which people decide to use services.

As discussed in the next two chapters, lay perspectives may involve other elements and types of rationalities which need to inform a research and policy agenda which seeks to understand the way in which people use services in the way they do and when they do. Additionally, there is a tendency for these models to view decision making for medical care in terms of a static framework. This is conceptualized as involving the making of choices from a range of possibilities at one point in time rather than as a process of ongoing contact over months or years, which is the pattern of health care use for a substantial number of people using primary care and other health services. Similarly extra-individual factors, 'group influence', or 'interpersonal networks' are viewed as an adjunct rather than being at the heart of decision making.

Help seeking as a social process forms a minority trend within the work undertaken in the area of health utilization behaviour. The potential of this approach lies in its ability to move beyond a focus on the individual, his or her symptoms, social and psychological profiles. More specifically it allows an identification of when and how people use services rather than identifying whether they have ever used them. The potential for identifying illness behaviour in community contexts using a variety of formal and informal health resources also holds out potential for applying it to the use of primary care services. Thus, the social process approach discussed at the end of this chapter goes some way to balancing the defects inherent in the 'individualistic' decision-making models. In the next chapter we develop elements of the social process approach by examining the relevance of the experience of illness and past use of services in influencing the formulation of demand at the interface between lay and primary care. This is then developed further in subsequent chapters where we look at other factors which influence the process of demand formulation, such as social interactions and networks; the informal provision of health care; the provision of health care through community pharmacy; and the availability of relevant information for accessing the most appropriate and effective health care.

NOTES

1 In support of this argument he refers to strong correlations between measures of 'neuroticism' or psychological distress and the number of symptoms reported on a symptom list.
2 It may be that in a climate of resource constraint the profession of medicine is more aware of the consequences of medicalization whereas medicalization may be viewed as less problematic when resources are not in short supply.
3 For instance, in relation to mental health service utilization, help seeking has been found to be associated with a wide range of factors including the stigma of seeking help; attitude towards services; treatment fearfulness; level of distress; gender; age; education; race; urbanization; and insurance coverage (Saunders 1993).
4 In this regard the extensive amount of sociological research undertaken into the relationship between paid and unpaid work and control over health can be viewed as a direct response to the inadequacies of locus of control health research (e.g. Muellen 1992; Bloor 1995; Rogers *et al.* 1998).

PART II

LAY ACTION IN THE FORMULATION OF DEMAND

4

HOW THE EXPERIENCE OF ILLNESS AND SERVICE USE SHAPES HELP SEEKING

Time past and time future
What might have been and what has been
point to one end, which is always present

(T. S. Eliott, Burnt Norton)

The propensity to consult primary care services can be understood both in terms of people's social situations and the meaning they give to health and illness. In measuring quality of life or satisfaction with health services, people's views about health and sickness are often separated off from action taken about illness and the wider context within which it is experienced (Bowling 1995). In this and subsequent chapters we attempt to draw out connections between people's conceptions of illness and their use of services, use of self, lay and community resources, and help seeking. As we noted in the last chapter, one of the deficiencies of approaches to the investigation of demand for health care has been the lack of understanding of the processes and reasons for use seen from the patient's perspective. The social process approach goes some way towards overcoming these limitations. The strength of this approach lies in its ability to shift the focus from individual choice to socially constructed decisions to consult. There are a number of components to this which need unpacking in more detail. In this chapter we explore the way in which the experience of illness and past service use shapes people's help-seeking behaviour.

There are a multiplicity of factors which shape our views and experiences of health and illness and health action. These relate to the way in which the subjective meaning of people's experiences and biographies are linked to wider social and economic circumstances, as well as the immediacy of health problems. Within medical sociology and health services research, there is a well-established tradition of examining lay explanations, understandings and experience of illness, and the way in which people interpret and read bodily signs and reactions in assessing illness (Fitzpatrick *et al.* 1986; Radley 1994). Tapping common-sense ideas has also been viewed as valuable for comprehending the way in which official health messages are assimilated and understood, and influence health action undertaken by individuals (Cornwell 1984; Davison *et al.* 1991; Backett 1992; Rogers and Pilgrim 1995). Blaxter (1985) takes the view that while lay concepts of health and illness are at times less 'expert' than professional views, because they are grounded in subjective experience, in other ways they may be better informed. Everyday 'lived experience' also provides an intimate taken-for-granted knowledge of the body in which individuals observe and reflect on signs and symptoms emotionally and cognitively. These form the basis of communications and action about health and illness (Olin Lauritzen 1997).

There are both similarities and differences between lay and medical constructions of health and illness. There has, at times, been a tendency to overemphasize the distinction between the two. However, expert and lay knowledge are mutually dependent in their formation and 'lay' cannot be seen as separate from medical knowledge. Common-sense knowledge is in part derived from, and incorporates, both expert and medical meanings. De Swaan (1990) has used the term 'proto-professionalization' to refer to the way in which lay understandings have become influenced by professional constructs of health and illness. Medical ideas and knowledge are made available to people from a variety of sources and these are incorporated into the way in which people think about and respond to episodes of illness. (These are examined in more detail in Chapter 8.) Here, we examine:

- the meaning and judgements people make about illness as the basis of lay people's help-seeking activities, and
- the way in which the experience and past use of primary care services can shape subsequent use.

THE CAUSE, MEANING, AND EVALUATION OF SYMPTOMS

Just as the process of diagnosing forms the basis of medical practice, in a similar way the views about the cause, prognosis and risk of symptoms form the basis of lay people's help-seeking activities. An understanding of the meaning of symptoms involves competing cognitions and perceptions. The meanings people attribute to symptoms provide one understanding of cues to health action. They also account in part for service utilization. Perceptions of health and illness have been viewed as being linked to the social and subjective contexts of people's everyday lives (Davison *et al.* 1991; Backett 1992; Castro 1995). A moral imperative ingrained in constructs of health and illness has also been linked to the use of services. A study by Williams (1983), for example, points to the high value attached to stoicism which is conducive to the toleration of, rather than help seeking for, symptoms. The way in which illness is construed also appears to have an impact on people's illness management strategies. Hertzlich and Piernet (1973) found that people who typified illness as an 'occupation', where there was an expressed need to fight and control the impact of illness, would do anything to seek medical care. Others who saw illness as a destructive force managed illness through denial and thus tended to avoid consultation.

Changes over time in the symbolic and cultural significance of symptoms may impact on both the way illness is experienced and action which is taken. In relation to help seeking for primary care the concept of tiredness is a good example. In his study of the process of becoming ill, Robinson (1971) noted that tiredness was consistently recognized in middle-class families as a sign of illness, but in working-class families there was a tendency towards accepting tiredness as a normal part of life. This in turn was linked in people's narratives and expectations about tiredness from undertaking manual work. Changing norms about the significance and meaning attached to tiredness as a symptom of illness are indicated by the fact that it is now one of the most common complaints made by patients to doctors in general practice and that it is recognized as occuring among patients in all social classes (Fitzgibbon *et al.* 1997).

THE RELEVANCE OF ENVIRONMENT AND SOCIAL POSITION TO PEOPLE'S NOTION OF THE CAUSES OF ILLNESS

The causes of illness identified by lay people have been considered relevant to the meanings people attribute to illness. In the 'Pathways to Care' study, the cause of problems sometimes provided a backdrop to the way in which individuals experienced service use. A questioning of the legitimacy of expressing a view about cause was

linked, particularly among elderly patients, to a reliance on, or deference to, medical authority in health matters: 'I thought the symptoms might have been connected in some way, but I mean I don't
know, I'm not that much of a medical specialist'. However, other
people were more forthcoming. As with other studies, there was evidence of the range of causes of illness which included reference to
genetic, biomedical and psycho-social causes of illness. For some
respondents the immediate environment and social position of
people informed the way in which they conceptualized their problems, and woven into some narratives were accounts of the causes of
health problems which were linked to living in a particular locality.

There was evidence in the accounts of some people of the multiple problems of deprivation and the drug problems on the estate
in the inner city location which formed one of the three areas in
which the 'Pathways to Care' study was conducted. Drug taking and
alcoholism in the area were seen to lead directly to physical problems such as liver failure and heart disease. They were also viewed
indirectly as a drain on health and social resources in the locality,
which could present difficulties for people in accessing health care.
(In this regard, one couple who had young children suggested that
there should be a separate building at the side of the surgery for 'the
addicts'.) A combination of high unemployment, being short of
money and working in untoward environments (e.g. the cold in
meat production factories), poor diet, and a 'lack of awareness',
were also cited as causative factors in a range of acute and chronic
illnesses. Discussing the cause of her daughter's asthma, this
account of a mother from a rundown and deprived area who had
recently been rehoused to another part of the estate illustrates the
connections people make between the locality, external environment and the internal living arrangements:

> We've got two motorways, you've got the aeroplanes coming
> over dropping all their crap over this estate, you can put your
> washing out and it's covered in fuel by morning...We were
> living in one of the tower blocks and water was just pouring
> down the walls ... with S having asthma it just wasn't on.

The woman went on to describe a lack of resources for children's
recreation and 'green spaces'. The extra runway planned for the
nearby airport she felt would compound the problems further.
There was a pessimism about the multiple problems which were felt
to be beyond amelioration, expressed in the view that the estate
should be 'demolished'.

In the rural locality, which was more affluent, narratives about the nature of the environmental and social problems and their connection with health problems were of a different order. In the poor and deprived area the causes of illness were related to a number of dimensions of deprivation in people's lives: housing, dampness, unemployment, and the presence of people with particular problems, (e.g. drug addicts) were among the ones most frequently mentioned. In contrast, in the more affluent and rural area there was a much greater focus on a *single* environmental cause – the emissions from two chimneys of a local cement factory were mentioned spontaneously by a third of the respondents in this locality. While this did not preclude a multi-causation view of illness, external causes were more likely to be viewed as part of a global problem affecting all areas, rather than located within the immediate circumstances of the everyday lives of people living in the area:

> *It's not a good area for bronchial chest disease. They don't like to admit it and they don't like to tell us, but there are two chimneys there which has got a lot to do with it.*

> *Well it's a damp area and I don't think that helps. I'm not saying it causes it, and people do blame the cement works, but then there's a lot of pollution in the area in general isn't there, from all over the world probably.*

The views that people held about the link between the cause of problems and the locality formed part of the context within which the threat of illness and symptoms were evaluated and illness managed.

EVALUATING SYMPTOMS AND THE ASSESSMENT OF RISK

Lay problem formulation is not an instantaneous process. It takes place over time and is likely to involve different levels of complexity depending on the nature and familiarity of the problem. In a recent study of depression, problems were found to have been formulated over a number of months. Problem recognition was found to be particularly difficult for the two groups who were most and least distressed, with the former reporting the most difficulty (Saunders 1993). Assessment of everyday health problems also takes place with reference to perceived stages in the life course and subjectively defined appropriateness of behaviour. Backett and

Davison (1995) found in their study on perceptions of health that illness assessment and avoidance emerge with new social expectations, experiences and responsibilities. The later life stages were overlain with normative and moral considerations such as having a partner, or taking on a mortgage and having children.

Behavioural cues judged against everyday normal behaviour form a significant part of the evaluation of symptoms. For example, mothers' intuition and close monitoring of children make them aware of subtle behavioural changes which are unlikely to be visible or significant to the medical expert (Cunningham-Burley 1990). For this reason parents may at times be more effective than professionals in the early diagnosis of a wide range of problems in their children. Assessing the nature of the cause of a problem is also relevant in deciding whether to deal with a problem oneself or seek external assistance. Where the cause of a problem is apparent, consultation is a less likely option than where it is not. Robinson (1971) found that decisions to seek formal help occurred where uncertainty arose in families over what was wrong and where difficulty was experienced in interpreting the seriousness of signs and symptoms. Similarly, in a study of cardiac patients urgent medical attention was considered to be necessary when pain was sudden, acute and unexpected (Cowie 1976). Most of the respondents initially attempted to normalize the experience by attributing a common-sense rather than a medical label, for example, they attributed pain to 'indigestion', or to other recent minor ailments. This process of 'normalization' was disrupted when the interpretive framework available failed to account for their experience.

These processes identified by previous studies were also evident in the accounts from individuals in the 'Pathways to Care' study. Making sense of the meaning and seriousness of bodily experiences, judged against a variety of possible and competing explanations for the presence of symptoms, was important in accounting for health actions that were taken. 'Feeling tired all the time' is one symptom associated with a range of conditions which can also be construed as nothing to do with illness or attributed to prescribe treatment. One man of 65 attributed his feelings of tiredness to a combination of age, his medical condition (angina) and the use of drugs. However, the fact that the tiredness was considered to be an obvious result of these factors meant that as a result of his own evaluation he had not sought attention for his symptoms from his doctor:

Well yes [long-term tiredness] but that's brought about by the, um, angina you know, beta blockers which slow your heart down, erm, so that, I mean if you are walking fast up a hill, something has to happen, normally your heart speeds up to cope with the extra energy required, now if you've got beta blockers that doesn't happen, your heart is limited at a certain speed, therefore your legs get tired to slow you down . . . don't forget that age comes into it as well.

The effect of drugs is a common reason given for feeling tired all the time. This makes the evaluation of the symptom of tiredness, separated off from the treatment prescribed, a difficult and uncertain task for patients and clinicians alike. The ability to contain symptoms and deal with them is also linked to thresholds of perceived risk and vulnerability. In addition to the immediacy of a problem, decisions to use services are made on the basis of what might happen if services are sought or not, rather than on an evaluation of existing behaviour or signs and symptoms of illness (Rogers 1990; Roberts 1992). In the 'Pathways to Care' study, risk to other people in the immediate household or family network was sometimes found to be the overriding reason for going to the doctor. In the case of this young woman, the threat her ear infection might pose to her husband's health was at least as important as the symptoms and duration of pain she was experiencing:

My husband is deaf so anything to do with ears – very obviously any infection that he might get really affects his hearing.

A mother with a young baby reported going to the GP when she was ill: 'to get it sorted out straight away' because she was afraid she would pass it on to the baby. Similarly, an elderly couple who reported infrequently consulting the doctor for themselves (other than for repeat prescriptions) despite a history of serious medical conditions, consulted the GP for a sore throat when they felt there was a danger of passing this onto their grandchildren:

I just go because of the grandchildren, they come here you see to the house, and it's no use sitting here with sore throats. You can pass it on . . . it isn't fair. I won't mess with the grandchildren.

Personal biography, familial culture, and the experience of illness over time, have also been shown to influence the way in which people make sense of and act upon symptoms.[1] This was evident in our study, with accounts which showed that lay symptom evaluation differed according to condition and personal experience. One woman talked about the way in which she assessed symptoms in her child with reference to 'knowing asthma' as a result of observing her brother and husband having asthma attacks. In her description she talked confidently and authoritatively about her evaluation and action:

> *Respondent:* *Well he [her son] has a happy wheeze, that means he's always happy so you can't diagnose when he's ill.*
> *Interviewer:* *How did you know to take him to the doctor's?*
> *Respondent:* *He's coughing, choking and I could really hear him wheezing. Normally when I give him the spray it calms down, the wheeze goes. And it didn't, so that was why I took him up [to out of hours services]. . . . I've got a problem with him having a happy wheeze – you can't always diagnose when they are ill and when they are not, you've just got to look out for it.*

Learning what to do about symptoms could also take place over a much shorter time span. One woman provided an account which illustrated how evaluating the significance and meaning of her first child's symptoms in one episode of illness quickly fed into the decision she took in relation to her second child who began to develop the same symptoms. The decision to go to the GP with her child was taken after six days, whereas the referral for the second child was decided upon immediately the symptoms appeared. Having bought cough medicine from the pharmacist for her first child's cough, she provided the following account:

> *Her cough didn't improve at all. Her throat was looking sore, and she was coughing. I rang the doctor. The actual thing is she'd go a day and all of a sudden she'd go into this like coughing bout, and it was just about tea time and she went into this coughing bout, and I could see like little red marks coming under her eyes and I thought, God what's that? You know, and that's when I rang the doctor . . . And he said well if she's no better bring her down in the morning and so the following day she's fine and then we went shopping. Going round Asda she had another attack with all this coughing you see. So come Monday that's when I took her down and he put her on antibiotics . . .*

The woman then went on to point to other cues about the nature of the illness which, together with her knowledge about her first child needing the GP, led to a quicker evaluation phase and response to the symptoms of her second child:

> *Since she's had the cough my friend's little one had had a really severe cough, you know what I mean? And like my mother-in-law, she's said that two little girls next door to her have had a very severe cough, as if there was a severe cough going round, because it's like she was going red in the face with it, but it was certain bouts which sounded a bit like whooping cough ... They have little bouts of it don't they and then when R [her second child] started I just noticed he was doing a few little coughs and I thought, Oh I'm getting him down straight away you know, and that's when I took him down because S she still had the cough after the antibiotics, you know what I mean?*

Other descriptions from the study illustrated the importance of different types of knowledge and authority in feeling able to make judgements about symptoms and what course of action should be subsequently taken. For example, there appeared to be a coalescence of lay and professional knowledge in the account of an evaluation of a nurse who went to her GP with an ear infection. Her evaluation of her health problem was derived from a combination of her training as a nurse, and the experience of living with her husband who had developed a hearing impairment. Her account of identifying an ear infection was more suggestive of a biomedical way of assessing signs and symptoms than some of the other accounts of similar health problems:

> *I had pain all down the side of my face one day and the next day I blew my nose and I went dizzy and my ear popped, so I thought that's what it is [ear infection].*

Judgements about symptom severity involve an assessment of what people are told about the nature of a condition from formal health service sources, their own personal experience, and other cues and information they may pick up informally. One woman who went to the doctor about her five-year-old daughter's stomach upset, provides an account of her and her partner's assessment of the situation. This in turn is overlain by the GP's reassurance, which is accepted but then comes under scrutiny because of observations and comments from others:

> *She goes to the toilet about five times a day, which they say can
> be quite normal, whatever. But you never know where you are
> with her, one minute you go in the morning and its runny, one
> minute you go and it's all right, then you go and it's not . . . he
> [the doctor] tries to assure me there is nothing wrong with her, I
> mean I'll give him that . . . so you come away thinking well they
> know best . . . but I don't know it's just [sighs], maybe that's
> probably all it is, I mean she's been like that since she was three
> years old, but I mean I speak to a lot of people at school and
> their kids don't go to the toilet five times a day . . .*

Expectations about health and the evaluation of symptoms in the
present are at times judged against early experiences and expectations. A man interviewed about his musculoskeletal problems,
who experienced repeated bouts of back pain from lifting awkwardly at work, reported visiting his doctor only four times over the
past fifteen years. He had not sought help from other sources and
considered himself to be in good health:

> *I was the seventh of eight children and born in the very very bad
> times and I'm talking now about 1925 and I was one of those
> people, it's a bit of a joke nowadays I suppose when people talk
> about it, but I was one of those people that suffered very badly
> at birth from rickets due to, so people tell me, from malnutrition
> . . . and when I was born I was so bow legged I couldn't walk. I
> was classed as a cripple but I had to wear rudimentary splints for
> certainly the first five and a half years, maybe six years; I still had
> them when I went to school. I used to have them on every night,
> just through the night not the day . . . I've been pleasantly sur-
> prised that I've come through so well . . .*

This last account is a good illustration of the way in which past
health problems can shape individuals' expectations about health in
the present. Another influence is the experience of using health
care services.

THE RELATIONSHIP BETWEEN PAST SERVICE
USE AND FUTURE USE

The experience of using services in the past appears to shape subsequent help-seeking behaviour. At times, direct service contact

has an obvious impact on subsequent use through the detection of illness by health care professionals (Miles 1991).[2] Another influence on subsequent use relates to the types of services and changes in availability of services. This connection is made by Williams (1983) in his study comparing lay logic in primary care consultations between Britain and France. French GPs were found to handle twice the rate of psychosomatic complaints than their British counterparts. Williams hypothesized that a capitation fee system (where a yearly 'lump sum' is paid for each patient) inhibits the expression of such illness compared with the impact on illness norms of a fee-for-service system. The impact of the experience of service use may also be transmitted rather than direct. Because people have ties to their social networks, negative or positive experiences have a 'ripple' effect to others by means of the 'stories' that are told about services and advice people give to others.

There are a number of specific elements of service delivery which are likely to influence the use of services. A personal long-term relationship with a practice or practitioner has been found to be a factor which patients rate highly. Satisfaction with care has been closely linked to the amount of time doctors spend with their patients and with opinions about their personal qualities (Eyles and Donovan 1990). Failure to seek medical help has been associated with disillusionment with professional help following contact with doctors who were unresponsive and unsympathetic (Scambler and Scambler 1984). The experience of service contact is likely to be structured according to who is doing the consulting. For example, one study has shown that Afro-Caribbean women's experience of working in health and welfare services informed the way in which they experienced services (Thorogood 1990). However, being treated civilly by health service professionals carried more importance and meaning for black women in the context of their experience of the response of health and welfare services to their needs more generally.

LEARNING WHAT TO DO FROM PREVIOUS CONSULTATIONS

An assessment of what can and cannot be done based on prior contact with services also appears to influence help seeking. Telles and Pollack (1981), for example, found that patients learned to fit into what was required of them from prior experience of what doctors considered to be a legitimate illness. In particular, patients learn to differentiate their feelings to the appropriate degree otherwise they risk not being treated or not receiving sick role legitimation. According to the authors, feeling sick and knowing how to use the health system involves 'a mutual influence ... in which the physician's knowledge shapes the individual's experience of illness and the individual's experience and social needs permit entry into the sick role – shape the physician's knowledge'.

This process is evident in a study of the management of cystitis in primary care, in which the nature of the experience feeds back into how women subsequently perceive and manage their symptoms (Pill 1987). Contact with the doctor enabled women to put a label on symptoms, but doctors' frequent use of the infection model and their emphasis on the random nature of the attacks tended to limit the control women felt they could exercise in managing their condition. This appeared to be compounded by a reported lack of information about the diagnosis that was being made. There was little attempt to elicit women's own ideas about what was wrong and little reinforcement of self-help measures. Thus the experience of seeing a doctor for an ailment at one point in time may increase the likelihood of future help seeking, as indicated by this quote from Pill (1987):

> Consultation means medication, with the result that women are often reinforced in the belief that the best strategy is to go to the doctor quickly and get the appropriate tablets, rather than delay and try self remedies.

A recent randomized controlled trial identified a similar process operating in relation to another common reason for consultation. Little *et al.* (1997) found that prescribing antibiotics for sore throats did little to alleviate symptoms but enhanced the belief in the efficacy of antibiotics. Patients given antibiotics were more likely to believe that they were effective and report an intention to consult in the future than patients who were not given them. These studies suggest that expectations are mutually constructed and reinforcing and are often doctor-initiated. The 'Pathways to Care' study also suggested that at times it was doctors' rather than patients' expectations that patients should have antibiotics. There was evidence of patients resisting an over-reliance on prescribing. A few respondents reported changing doctors because of 'pill pushing': 'I changed doctors because I didn't like the way he was giving out antibiotics willy nilly'.

The interview data from the pathways study also elaborated on the processes and subtle ways in which use and contact for one problem can influence the way in which people continue to seek help or do so for other ailments in the future. In some cases this constituted the straightforward following of advice when next contacting services. This mother got in touch with the out-of-hours advice service after following advice she had previously been given:

> *Interviewer:* How did you get his temperature down?
> *Respondent:* Err Calpol and a wet flannel. I'd already done that anyway, but it hadn't come down.
> *Interviewer:* Right.
> *Respondent:* But erm, they just said, keep giving him it, whatever, I think it was every four hours and I just kept sponging him down.
> *Interviewer:* Is that what they told you to do?
> *Respondent:* We'll I'd done that anyway.
> *Interviewer:* And you explained that you'd done that anyway?
> *Respondent:* Yeah, just carry on doing it.
> *Interviewer:* How did you know to do that?
> *Respondent:* Well I'd been told before by the doctors.
> *Interviewer:* Right, what to do?
> *Respondent:* Yeah.

Learning that the doctor will respond to some symptoms and not others was also evident in the evaluation of symptoms by another mother of young children who explained: 'I don't take the children to the GP if they have "bright eyes", because the GPs don't bother as long as they are bright eyed.' She would take the children to the GP, however, if *'they get really poorly and don't want to do anything'*.

A more complex interaction of expectation, prior experience and contact with service also emerged from people's narratives. This included in-depth knowledge about the workings of the referral system and knowledge about the scarcity and availability of resources for treating a particular problem. For example, one woman who had previously had a helpful period of counselling, on experiencing feelings of anxiety following a divorce went straight-away to the GP, and on the third visit the issue of referral for counselling was discussed:

So I approached him quite early on ... well, he asked my opin-
ion, if I would like some counselling and I'd already seen X
before two years ago when my marriage was ending, when we
were separating, so I said 'yes, I would like to speak to X
again ...'. I approached him early because I knew that even
though I was being referred I would have a very long wait
because the previous time I had to wait six months before I was
referred. I thought it would be better to do it right away rather
than wait until I was at my wits' end and then still have a long
wait. That's another reason why I did it early.

In contrast, a woman who described herself as having poly-arthritis
which regularly flared up, causing severe pain and swelling of joints,
rarely used services because of learning the limits of what formal
services have to offer. This coalesced with her formulation of her
illness as predetermined:

Interviewer: So in between, if your pains get worse, do you
bother coming back [to the doctor]?

Respondent: Well no, not with the arthritis, no, because I feel
there is nothing else they can do. The chiropractor
and doctor said to me, it won't go away. Like with
the arthritis I know that there isn't much more they
can do with that ... Well it's just one of them
things, it's hereditary, it's in the family ... my
mum's grandma was doubled up with it. She
couldn't do nothing for herself. She was in a
wheelchair, she had to be put in and out of bed,
undressed and things like that. And they say it was
third generation or something which came down
to me. So I've got everything, I get everything me.

There were other ways in which contact with primary care set the
parameters of the kind of help and the way in which help should
subsequently be sought for a problem. At times this amounted to
a need to exploit one option before trying another. A woman who
had a sore and bent finger which was not getting better reported
not taking her husband's advice to seek alternative help and
refused to return to the GP for more help because of the understood expectation of finishing treatment before requesting further
assistance:

I went to the doctor's; I think he was pretty vague, he didn't know
if it was one thing or the other. So he said, 'We'll start with the

*anti-inflammatory tablets', which is a course which seems to go
on forever, and my husband keeps saying to me, 'Why don't you
go to the osteopath?', and I say, 'No, I'll finish with the doctor's
first', but I haven't finished my pills so I know he'll only say to
me, 'Well you haven't finished your course', but I've only got
four or five days to go now so then I'll make an appointment. . .'*

THE IMPACT OF CONTACT ON SUBSEQUENT
HELP SEEKING

Negative prior contact with services has the potential to exacerbate unmet need, by reinforcing a reluctance to use services when
they are required, and raises questions about the quality of care
that is received once contact has been made. An example of this
was suggested by a young family with multiple health problems.[3]
Both adult members reported using the doctor as little as possible
and this was based on their previous negative experience of use of
services relating to misdiagnosis and learning the limits of
medicine in relation to previous consultations. Here, a woman in
her thirties describes her contact with primary care for her back
problem:

Respondent: *I wasn't diagnosed for nine years, and at one stage
they [the GPs] more or less wiped their hands of
me and said, 'There's nothing wrong with you, it's
all in your mind, go away', and when my husband
went and had discussions, shall we say, they said,
'Oh we've got what we call compassion fatigue,
because she's been ill for so long we have no compassion left', that's what they said. My husband
went to see my GP. He was there for an hour and
a half. And they said, 'Well there's nothing wrong
with you, go away, it's all in your mind', so my
husband turned round and said, 'Well if it's all in
her mind send her to a psychiatrist', 'Oh no we
wouldn't do that, we don't think it's that serious',
and then it was just a catalogue of nightmares and
then finally I had a second MRI [Magnetic Reson-
ance Imaging] scan.*

Interviewer: *So they found nothing on the first one?*

Respondent: *No, because they scanned the wrong part of my*

> *body, so when they did the second they discovered this problem.*

Another example of a prior negative encounter leading to a decrease in service use, despite perceptions on the part of this family of ongoing unresolved health problems, is provided by this woman's account of her husband's reluctance to use the GP:

> *He won't go [to the GP]. I literally have to drag him to get him to go. If he goes he seems to get fobbed off, he never comes away with a satisfactory answer. You know, 'Oh well you've got irritable bowel syndrome, take bran', you know, but no tests were done. He has hard lumps on his body that we believe are just benign cysts but no tests have ever been done, he's just been told, 'Oh they are nothing, go away.' And he worries about it, with all the cancer scares and goodness knows what else and he actually passed a kidney stone last week because he suffers from kidney stones, but he wouldn't go to the doctor's because he said, 'Oh no, I'll just be sent away, they won't do anything'.*

Evident in this last account is the transferability of the impact of a consultation for one condition when considering going to primary care for another. 'Fobbing off' may not always be a good demand management or reduction strategy (although arguably, in the above case, because the man didn't bother the GP again, it might have been viewed in this way, particularly given that irritable bowel syndrome is increasingly being considered an illness that can be treated by OTC (over the counter) medication or self-care). However, the failure to resolve a problem from a patient's viewpoint may result in *more* rather than fewer consultations. In the example below, a woman who felt she had not had the appropriate tests (for an arrythmia)[4] and was not reassured by her doctor's investigation of the complaint, consulted with another GP in the hope of gaining reassurance:

> Respondent: *I was expecting to be sent to have this kind of check-up that my brother had had in Israel. He'd had a really thorough examination, all day he was in there; he was monitored and they had him on the bike and I was expecting a similar sort of thing.*
> Interviewer: *We're you right and what actually did happen?*
> Respondent: *Not a lot. She sort of said, 'Well really there is nothing for you to worry about. I'm not saying there's nothing wrong because obviously there is,*

> *but what I'm saying is it's not cause for concern',*
> *but she seemed to think it was a bit difficult to*
> *know what to do next . . . and she sort of said, the*
> *difficulty is knowing what to do next or what steps*
> *to take. Let's start with an ECG. When I went back*
> *it was like, 'Oh nothing showed up on your ECG,*
> *you're obviously quite fit, your blood pressure is*
> *all right, your cholesterol is all right', and she said*
> *just carry on with what you are doing . . .*

Interviewer: *And have you spoken to her about it since?*

Respondent: *Well what happened, I had to go again, a couple*
> *of weeks ago because I had a bit of a bad chest . . .*
> *so I went to see a different doctor deliberately*
> *because there's this doctor there that nobody wants*
> *to see, because she's a swine, but I thought well . . .*
> *So I went to see her and I just said, 'Oh by the*
> *way, while I'm here I'm just a bit concerned, . . .*
> *and she just said there's nothing at all to worry*
> *about.*

Interviewer: *And what prompted you to actually go?*

Respondent: *I think I just wanted more reassurance.*

Interviewer: *Oh so it wasn't really your chest?*

Respondent: *No that was on its way out. I'd treated it with oils*
> *all week.*

In another instance, a young woman who had originally gone to the GP with a problem about her mouth ended up, after extensive investigations seeing two different dentists and using homeopathic medication. A failure to accept the outcome of the initial investigation and formulation of the problem was compounded by a lack of information. The perceived fatalistic attitude of her GP left this woman searching for a more positive direction to prevent her problems getting worse:

> *The GP said, 'We'll put you down for you to get a prescription*
> *for this artificial saliva which is just a spray in your mouth' . . . I*
> *said to my husband, 'They went into all this scanning and things*
> *and all I want is my mouth back to normal.' I've been to two*
> *dentists because I thought maybe my dentist got it wrong. I*
> *think, when he [the GP] gave me that artificial saliva he said*
> *about me having arthritis in the neck, and I said, 'Well, well what*
> *do we do about that then?' He said, 'Well you've got pain*
> *killers.' And I said, 'Well what can I do to prevent it getting any*

worse?' And he went, 'Nothing really', and that was that. But I thought, 'Well I want to know if there is anything you can do. Like I said to my mate, 'You see old people and they have little crinkled up hands with arthritis and it's in my neck. Am I ending up like that? And I thought, Is there nothing like cod liver oil or something like that that you should take? And he said, 'No, once it's there it's there.' So I thought that was a bit off, that's why I went to the homeopath.

The limited and appropriate use of diagnostic tests is an accepted part of good evidence-based practice. However, the understanding and meaning of tests may hold a different significance for patients. In the following example the failure to address the reasons behind a patient's desire for an X-ray for musculoskeletal pain resulted in a subsequent call for a home visit:

Respondent: I mean I suppose I can't blame the doctor because they knew what it was, but I was a little bit annoyed to think that they wouldn't let me have an X-ray to see ... I wasn't sleeping with it and I thought I'd ring and I asked the doctor to come out to me, and it was one of the lady doctors that came, and I said, 'I can't go on with this much longer. Can't you send me anywhere for an X-ray?' 'No', she said, 'no, we know what it is and it's just a matter of time.' Well it was, it was so long, it was unbelievable really ...

Interviewer: How did you think an X-ray might have helped?

Respondent: Well I just thought, to be honest I'll tell you something now, I really thought it was a lot more severe than it was. I thought literally at one point I was dying, it was that bad ... I was in absolute agony. I mean I'm not a mard person by any means but I was nearly in tears with it all the time really.

She felt the severity of the pain was not appreciated by the doctor, nor was the diagnosis the doctor provided an acceptable one:

Well all I get is, 'It's your age.' It seems to be everything that is wrong with you today, it's your age. Well I thought it was something to do with the fall, but no when I've asked him, he said, 'No, it's an old age thing.' I said, 'Well I'm not that old, I mean I don't feel that old ...

In contrast to the experience of consulting with the GP, the physio-therapist was felt to be much more emphatic and effective. This was attributed to his own personal experience of back pain, the explanation given of the cause of the pain (a trapped nerve) and instruction about rest and exercise. These were reassuring and a persuasive way of managing the problem, although the woman's expectations of recovery were modest.

Although, fatalism about a condition was one message people internalized from contact with services, a different response from primary care could result in a more satisfactory outcome for the patient. An account from this elderly woman with chronic pain, who was initially reluctant to contact services again because she thought nothing more could be done, indicates a meeting of need when her doctor tried using acupuncture:

> *The pain was so bad, err, I mean I would be doing this [wincing]. L [her husband] would say, 'For goodness sake K stop it', and I'd say, 'Well, I'm sorry, but the pain is so bad', so he kept on at me. So after two years I said, 'All right, to keep the peace I'll go back to the doctor's.' So I went back and saw him and I said, 'There's nothing you can do for my knee is there?' and he said 'Well no, you were lucky not to lose your leg really', and then he suddenly said to me, 'Look, would you like to try acupuncture? Dr C does it. You can have it because you are in the practice.' So I said, 'Yes please', you know, you'll try anything when you are in pain, so I went to him and he said to me, 'Well I can't guarantee anything, it may be worse after the first one.' It wasn't actually, and I had, I think about eight and the pain went like that. It gradually got less. After the second it started to get better, I said to him, 'I'm frightened to say this to you, but it is a bit better', and after about four he said, 'well, we'll leave it a fort-night instead of a week'. I used to go once a week, but after a week the pain came back you see, so then after eight it was fine. Now he said to me, 'Now I don't know how long this will last but as soon as you get pain again you ask to come and see me again.' It lasted for three months and so then I made an appointment. I went back and I had two more and that is three years ago.*

Indirectly, information and perceptions about the changes in the organization and delivery of primary care services can also impact on the way in which people use services. A man with a long history of manic depression reported limiting his contact with his GP to no more than twice a year and never for his mental health problem.

This, he reported, was due to fears of being removed from the doctor's list. The need to ration his use of services was set against the information he had gleaned from newspapers about a cash-strapped NHS. Additionally, he was mindful that his status as a psychiatric patient may make him liable for removal from his doctor's list.

The appointment system operated by primary care services is also relevant to decision making. Appointments, in theory, should make access to services easier by specifying a time that is convenient for the patient. The experience of some people in this study is that this sometimes does not happen and this feeds back into the way in which people deal with their problems. An example of the imperative of work routines fitting in with illness was provided by a woman who ran a nursing home. She had a bent swollen finger. Having been to the GP once she needed a return visit, but found it difficult to plan her work to fit in with an appointment several days hence:

> *Because of the domiciliary [visit] I have to do . . . when you ring the doctor's, they will give you an appointment and it might be like next week. Well you don't know what you're going to be doing next week. Because of the domiciliary, we've got to go mornings, afternoons, you know, whatever . . . Yeah, it's to do with the home . . . I mean like now, if I rang up and they said, 'Oh yes, we'll see you at 5pm today', well fine, I'll be OK today at 5.00 p.m. but next week, this time at 5.00 p.m. I won't know what I'm doing.*

There are a number of questions that are raised by these accounts. First, there is the issue of whether it is reasonable for people to expect to be able to do something positive about long-term chronic illnesses. Second, is it the responsibility of services to work with patients' own expectations and desires rather than expect patients simply to take away and be satisfied with the message that they are given? People, as we will see from Chapter 6, are willing to try a range of options and often make strenuous efforts at self-care and alternative care. One of the questions that is raised is the extent to which services and professionals have the capacity to work with patient-led agendas with a view to managing the demand for health services better.

SUMMARY

In this chapter the focus has been on the way in which individual conceptions and experiences of health and illness are likely to be important factors in health care utilization. A number of factors including the immediate locality, familial history and past individual experiences of illness form the backdrop to expectations and health actions in seeking care from primary care services. Similarly the experience of using services, including negative experiences and learning the limits of what can be provided, influences the use of services even at times where the need for health care may be significant. The nature of contact with services is crucial to an understanding of the formulation of subsequent demand. Dissatisfaction with services or professional attitude may fail to meet patient need and thus exacerbate it. Some people may then be reluctant to use services for a problem they have been told is untreatable. Others may consult *more* in an attempt to gain needed help, reassurance or problem resolution. Conversely, alternative ways of responding may lead to better problem resolution for some people which may negate the necessity to use services again. Thus, this analysis suggests that the type of service organization and response to patients seeking help from primary care may have a sustained impact on the way in which people formulate demand for future health care.

Other aspects of the social process of help seeking will be explored in the next chapter. The focus is on examining the processes of help seeking which flow on from the recognition of illness which has been discussed in the first part of this chapter. The impact of social ties or networks on help-seeking behaviour and the relevance of the way in which others construe health and illness will be investigated.

NOTES

1 The extent of 'worry' about an illness episode has been linked to personal experience of severe disease in respondents' family histories (Borosson and Rastam 1993) and the propensity to consult has been related to different childhood experiences and perceptions of the way in which illness is managed in adults' families when they were children (Weich *et al.* 1996).

2 For example, it has been hypothesized that the difference in consultation rates for hypertension between men and women is due to the fact that the blood pressure of women is more frequently taken as part of antenatal care and prescriptions for oral contraceptives and hormone replacement therapy.

3 At the time of the interview the man was deaf, had had a stroke and renal failure in the past and had continuing ear and chest infections. The

woman had a past history of skin allergies and had had severe back problems which had necessitated the removal of two vertebrae in her spine. Her daughter was asthmatic.

4 Knowledge of the tests undergone by her brother for the same complaint (heart arrythmia) led to her expectations for the full range of tests to be carried out.

5

THE INFLUENCE OF INDIVIDUALS' ACTION AND SOCIAL NETWORKS ON HELP SEEKING

The quality of life in the community and the extent to which people respect and support each other can (also) be important to our health. Social exclusion can have damaging health consequences.

(Department of Health, *Our Healthier Nation*)

In the previous chapter we explored the impact on help seeking of people's evaluation, experience of illness, and past use of services. In people's everyday lives the processes of recognizing illness and managing are not clearly demarcated. Episodes of illness and wellness draw on a wealth of previous experience and knowledge about illness, experience which is derived from family agendas, as well as previous contact with health services and interactions with professionals. Information sources and care provided by other individuals, informal sources and intermediaries are also relevant to the formulation of, and response to, illness. These processes are explored in this chapter and Chapters 6–8.

Out of all the models and approaches assessed in Chapter 3, the social process approach was the only one which stressed the importance of social interaction and social networks in making decisions to seek help. Hence this approach can contribute to an understanding of the variety of ways in which individuals use health care services. In this chapter we therefore make explicit the role played by individuals and other lay people in help seeking by concentrating on the combination of actors and types of interaction taking place before contact is made with formal primary care. In the first part of the chapter we present analyses of the different patterns of help seeking evident from our study of recent primary care use, and examine the way in which individuals contain illness as a phase prior to formal help seeking. In the second part of the chapter we draw together previous literature and further findings from our study in examining the processes involving individuals and others in mediating help seeking.

PATTERNS OF HELP SEEKING FOR PRIMARY CARE

The following preliminary results are based on data from the feasibility study 'Pathways to Care'.[1] The data come from the household interview and the four-week health diary. Information about the experience of illness, self-care and formal health care within the household was recorded in a structured diary on a daily basis. It is therefore possible to identify episodes of illness and relate these to health care actions. An illness episode is defined as a block of one or more consecutive days on which the respondent has experienced the same illness.[2]

The four-week health diaries were completed for 518 individuals of all ages (215 households). About half of these individuals had experienced one or more illness episodes, ranging from minor ailments such as a cold to more serious conditions such as heart problems. A large proportion of illnesses were minor – more than a third of all illnesses were reported as colds and 'flu.

About 250 people experienced a total of more than 500 illness episodes within the four-week period. Just over 110 of these illness episodes resulted in contact with formal health care services, of which about 100 were with primary care services.[3] This result is similar to White's study where 20 per cent of all symptoms and illnesses occurring within a month led to professional care (White *et al.* 1961). A health diary study carried out in Denmark also found that one out of four to five illness episodes in a 27-week period led to some kind of professional care (Bentzen *et al.* 1989).

In addition to professional care, we can also link other types of health actions to illness episodes. Information about self-care activities was also collected in the health diaries. Self-care was defined as changes in daily activities because of an illness or injury (i.e. staying at home from work or school, staying in bed, changing their diet/eating habits, using an aid or appliance) or taking non-prescribed remedies/medicines (i.e. home remedies, herbal products, homeopathic medicines and over-the-counter medicines). About 70 per cent of all illness episodes involved some form of such self-care activities.

We have classified illness episodes based on whether they involved self care and/or professional health care:

- no health action was reported for 24 per cent of illness episodes,
- only self-care activities were reported for 54 per cent of illness episodes,
- self-care activities and professional health care were reported for 17 per cent of illness episodes,
- only professional health care was reported for about 5 per cent of illness episodes.

It is interesting to note that only a small proportion of contacts with a health care professional did not involve some level of self-care.

The average length of an illness episode was about seven days. However, the average length differed significantly between those who did not report any health action, those who reported self-care activities but no professional care and those who reported professional care with or without self-care activities: two days, 4–5 days and 8–9 days respectively. The length of an illness episode may be an indicator of the seriousness of the illness or an indicator of the increasing impact the illness may be having on the person's life.

We have also applied logistic regression to identify factors which influenced the use of professional care. It should be noted, however, that our feasibility study is small and some degree of caution should be exercised when interpreting the results.

All adults aged 16 and over who had experienced one or more illness episodes in the four-week period have been included in the analysis (N = 176). As the individual is the analytic unit, illness episodes have been aggregated by individual. The dependent variable is whether an individual had used professional health care in the four-week period (with or without self-care). The independent variables included in the model are age; sex; number of illness days; whether the person had a limiting long-term illness; smoking status; whether the person had ever used alternative therapies; marital status; employment status; education; housing tenure; and whether the household received benefits. Given the exploratory nature of the analysis, the model was kept as simple as possible, i.e. only main effects and no interactions were fitted. The results of the model are presented in Table 5.1 and are expressed in terms of odds ratios.[4]

The only three factors which have a statistically significant effect

Table 5.1 Odds ratios of seeking professional health care: adults aged 16 and over who had experienced one or more illness episode in a four-week period (N = 176)

Independent variables	Odds ratios
Age	0.99
Sex	1.70*
(Female = 1)	
Number of illness days in four-week period	1.12*
Limiting long-term illness	1.09
(Yes = 1)	
Smoking status	1.25
(Yes = 1)	
Ever used alternative therapies	0.89
(Yes = 1)	
Area	
(C = 0)	
Br	1.21
B	0.92
Marital status	
(Single = 0)	
Married or cohabiting	2.01*
Widowed, divorced or separated	1.12
Employment status	0.77
(Employed = 1)	
Higher education	0.88
(Degree, professional/educational/vocational qualification = 1)	
Housing	1.11
(Rented accommodation = 1)	
Benefits	1.11
(Income support, family credit or housing benefit = 1)	

5 per cent significance level

are: sex, number of illness days and marital status. The odds of a woman using professional health care when ill was 1.70 times the odds of a man, holding the effects of the other variables constant. For each additional day of being ill there was a 12 per cent increase in the chance of using professional health care (again, holding the effects of the other variables constant). Those who were married were twice as likely as those who were single to seek professional health care (again, holding the effects of the other variables constant).

In conclusion, these preliminary results show that ill people are far more likely to use self-care than professional health care services. Also, the data suggest that people tend to wait some time before contacting a health care professional to treat their illnesses. When they do use professional health care, this tends to be in addition to self-care practices. Women are at higher risk of using professional health care than men. Compared to single people, those who are married or cohabiting are more likely to use professional health care.

THE CONTAINMENT OF ILLNESS

Implicit in the presentation of the data above is the importance, for undertaking health care and evaluating symptoms, of the timing between the onset of a problem and consultation. This is often not recognized by formal service providers and a lack of understanding or bewilderment is sometimes expressed when patients claiming to be ill have not consulted services when they have had the 'opportunity' (e.g. why do they consult out-of-hours services when they could have used daytime services?). The temporalizing of symptoms refers to the time between the onset of a problem and consultation. This can be for lengthy periods. A study about depression reported the time between onset and entering treatment as eight months (Monroe *et al.* 1991). As we discussed in the last chapter, part of this time 'lag' is usually taken up with recognizing and formulating the problem. However, even after the identification of a problem there is often still a significant time lag before formal support is sought, when individuals contain or deal with signs and symptoms in a variety of ways.

Matching the meaning that illness has for an individual with the action he or she subsequently takes has been approached within the social sciences in a number of different ways. From a psychoanalytically informed approach, motivations, meaning and responses to illness reflect hidden unconscious need to 'repress' or avoid dealing with the consequences of being ill. Waitzkin and Magana (1997), for example, have suggested that extreme stress 'is processed psychologically as a terrible, largely incoherent narrative of events too awful to hold in consciousness'. This, they argue, leads to the somatization of symptoms which are less threatening and more manageable for people to deal with. Other interpretations suggest,

for example, that cognitive representations of a problem will provide a meaning that allows individuals to consider and select suitable coping strategies (Leventhal and Nerenz 1985). People's
everyday social situations also affect the way in which they contain
symptoms and their ability to do so. With regard to the latter,
Alonzo (1984) has suggested that people contain symptoms within
a range of social situations influenced by a number of factors,
including:

• commitment to and engrossment in situations,
• tolerance given by others,
• power relationships among participants,
• coping resources of the situations,
• symptom meaning,
• the presence of normal processes and chronic diseases,
• age and sex as circumstances.

From this perspective, containment measures include strategies
such as suppressing signs and symptoms, ignoring them, concealing
them, or attending to them. These strategies are linked to particular types of situation influencing the probability of symptoms occurring. Thus in everyday activities such as reading, travelling to work,
family meals, the situations are not usually associated with the likelihood of symptoms occurring. In other situations expectations of
symptoms arising are greater: for example, high-risk occupational
settings, professional and amateur sports or during periods of
increased workload. Moving along the continuum of containment
to an illness state are 'in between' situations where signs and symptoms may break through the normality of everyday situations. This
might include the taking of psychotropic medication for exams,
resting briefly or taking painkillers. A number of factors in the
environment also influence action in containing symptoms. These
include bodily sensations affected by engrossment in and commitment to the situation; the meaning and evaluation of a person's
state by another person; the power of others in situations; and
resources available (e.g. access to pain killers) to manage symptoms. According to Alonzo (1984), when there is a decline in the
ability to contain signs and symptoms over a significant proportion
of this 'situation set', people are likely to resort to external sources
for assistance.

Alonzo's analysis resonates with the way in which people use
contemporary primary care services. A recent study (Punamaki

and Kokko 1995b) found that a significant minority of people consulted primary care services because symptoms were causing disruptions to daily activities and they required medical confirmation of their symptoms to enable them to take more time off work. People decided they would consult if their symptoms deteriorated or developed in certain ways. As we discussed in the last chapter, in making illness claims and seeking legitimation from others (including health professionals) individuals go through a process of *proving* they have feelings which represent sickness.

Work and the containment of illness

Past research suggests that people's involvement with work is important in shaping the way in which people deal with illness and use services. The perceived interference of symptoms with work performance can operate as a trigger to medical consultation. At other times, work may act to prevent the seeking of help. In Bloor's study of illness behaviour (1985), he found that residents sought to guard their work routines against disruption by illness. Similarly, Cowie (1976) found that a number of the people he had interviewed who had experienced a myocardial infarction attempted to complete routine work tasks in which they were engaged when their heart attacks were happening.

Exemplars from our research illuminate aspects of the self-evaluation and containment of symptoms phase. Both paid and unpaid work contexts shaped the way in which people contained symptoms or sought help from others. The capacity to manage symptoms is in part related to the type of work one is expected to do, combined with the type of symptom a person is experiencing. One woman, who subsequently was diagnosed as having ulcerative colitis, found that her gastrointestinal symptoms prevented the maintenance of an appropriate containment strategy in her job as a barmaid:

> *I'd been at work, but then I had to have three weeks off work because I couldn't cope with it. Working behind a bar I couldn't work with the symptoms, serving, and I'd thought, Oh my God it's coming, it was that bad. Once it did come and I thought, Oh, it's so embarrassing, and I nearly died a death, I had a week off and then I went back and then I had to come off two more weeks and then it was easing off, but it hadn't gone so I kept going back [to the doctor's].*

In some instances the need to maintain a viable work situation was more important than the distress or discomfort of dealing with the symptoms of illness. One 'bottom line' was the threat of the loss of a job. Previous research has indicated that people take into account their position in the labour market when they face the dilemma of whether or not to enter the sick role (Virtanen 1994). Here a nurse describes the way in which her job situation delayed the seeking of formal help after having a period off work with a back injury:

> *So I had four months off work and then went back and I did another three years, kept quiet about it, never said anything, because I was frightened of losing my job.*

A further example was of a woman who needed to work another year to get her pension. She looked after elderly and disabled people. The symptoms of asthma from which she periodically suffered posed a threat to this goal. The need to maintain her job and keep her symptoms at bay was an uphill struggle. In this context coping with work becomes the major problem that needs to be actively managed as symptoms impinge more and more onto the ability and capacity to carry out tasks and everyday work routines. Here the woman describes the deployment of personal coping resources which are needed to do this and how eventually, when these are exhausted, she resorts to going to the GP:

> *It's like working, I have to come home from work and go to bed. I have to come home and go straight to bed so I'm OK for the next morning. And at the weekend I've got to sleep all weekend so I can cope with going back to work on Monday. I just woke up one morning and I thought, This is silly. I'll go and see the GP again. He [the GP] said, 'Come off work.'*

Understanding the pressures associated with the need to maintain ordinary work routines provides a different context within which to understand a stoical attitude to illness which has been associated with a delay, or reluctance in seeking help from formal services (Williams 1983). There are costs in moving from a productive working role to one of consuming health care. Not only might stoicism be tied up with a moral view about the need to contain symptoms, it may also be related to the pragmatism of sustaining everyday routines, the material resources associated with being employed and the expectations set up by the conditions of work. This was evident in some people's biographical accounts when explaining their reluctance to use contemporary GP services:

> Respondent: *Well can I start at the beginning and say that I am one of those people that has to be dying before I went to see the GP.*
>
> Interviewer: *Why is that?*
>
> Respondent: *Well really it was because I was married in 1949 and had four children, the last of which was born in 1960, and I was the only one working and I had to keep six people so if I felt ill I went to work because at the start there was no family allowance or anything like that and basically no sickness [benefit]. People don't appreciate it but I left a damn big firm in 1975 and if you were a manual worker then in 1975, which is only 20 years ago, you didn't get a penny sick pay, you just had basic Department of Health social security, so basically I had to be dying before I would stay off work quite frankly.*

Symptom containment was also a feature of the pressing need to fulfil the routine tasks associated with child care and domestic work. One young mother who had a paid night job and looked after her two-year-old child during the day accommodated her symptoms (very bad headaches) rather than returning to the GP despite a gradual worsening of pain over a lengthy period of time.

> Respondent: *... what I try to do is pass it off because I'm cleaning up and I've J and you just don't think about it. But if I sit down at night I hold my head in my hands and it's, Oh God it's here again.*
>
> Interviewer: *So how do you manage, what do you do in the day?*
>
> Respondent: *Well through the day I persevere with it ... I'm running around, I've got a two-year-old ... I'm clearing up, cooking tea and things ... but at night they'll go to bed and if it gets really bad I'll take two or three [pain killers] and I'll go to bed.*

Formal service contact or contact with others may bring an end to ways in which individuals have accommodated symptoms. This is illustrated with reference to this man who carried on working despite having angina until the intervention of his GP:

> Interviewer: *So how did it affect your work life then?*
>
> Respondent: *It didn't.*

> *Interviewer:* Did you still carry on working and everything?
> *Respondent:* Yeah, I still carried on working.
> *Interviewer:* Until the last six months and then you were off ill
> with your heart again?
> *Respondent:* ... Anyway when I went to the doctor he said,
> 'How old are you?', and I told him, and he said,
> 'Oh well you've done enough', and that was it. I
> finished work on that basis ...

However, accessing the GP for help did not necessarily imply the abandonment of pre-existing attempts at self-help. Coping strategies continued after the person had presented a problem to the GP. When asked about what this middle-class woman did while on the waiting list to see a counsellor she said:

> *Just work, yes, I worked on my garden. I'm self-sufficient for vegetables and milk and eggs. I have this smallholding and it takes an awful lot of work to keep it going. Just, one person, so I just threw myself into that.*

This last point brings us onto considering the importance of other people in the processes and outcome of help-seeking behaviour. While individual action is clearly important in containing and coping with illness and making decisions about the use of services, the impact of other people in shaping illness behaviour, help seeking and pathways to care is also relevant.

THE INFLUENCE OF SOCIAL NETWORKS ON HELP SEEKING

Interaction in social networks forms the mechanisms through which individuals recognize health problems, contact health facilities, and comply with medical advice. Studies examining social networks have been concerned with the investigation of social linkages as a way of understanding people's actions. The notion of a 'social network' has been used as an analytic concept by social scientists to interpret behaviour in a wide variety of social situations (Bott 1971; Walker *et al.* 1977). Indeed, it has been suggested that it is useful to think of a social network as a set of personal contacts through which people maintain their social identity and receive emotional support, material aid, services information and new social contacts (Walker *et al.* 1977). In relation to help seeking for services, the concept of the lay referral system in which lay networks are viewed as having the capacity to act as a cultural resource of knowledge, advice and support controlling individual health action has been influential (Freidson 1970; McKinlay 1972; Pescosolido 1992). This network may include relatives, friends, neighbours, fellow employees.[5] Some, but not all, of those who make up a person's social network maintain relationships with each other, and these relationships will vary in many ways, depending, for example, on their intensity or frequency. Pescosolido (1992), who links a symbolic interactionist tradition with network theory, argues that when deciding whether or not to consult a doctor, people's decisions are affected by day-to-day interaction with other people. She suggests that people's attempts to cope with symptoms are affected by negotiation with others, while at the same time constrained by social structure (such as class or ethnicity). Thus Pescosolido (1992: 1109) asserts that 'Individuals are neither puppets of some abstract structure nor calculating individuals; people both shape and are shaped by social networks.'

Specific dimensions of networks related to help seeking include both their structure (i.e. the number, strength and type of ties) and their function (i.e. advice, material aid, emotional support). In terms of *size* some researchers have found that large friendship networks tend to encourage the use of professional services, while large family networks tend to support self-reliance (Salloway and Dillon 1973). The combination of *membership* (e.g. kin, friends) of a network is relevant to the levels of advocacy and social support which are provided (Auslander and Litwin 1990) as is *interconnectedness, activity and maturity of networks*. Close-knit networks have been associated both with longer delays in contacting services (Birkel and Repucci 1983) and more ready use of services (Bleeker *et al.* 1995). Proximity of network members has a complex and changing relationship to utilization. For example, McKinlay (1972) found that those who underutilized antenatal services were more likely than utilizers to be living with their family. However, more recent studies highlight the importance of telephone contact for maintaining long-distance family ties, and for providing social support,[6] suggesting that proximity may not in certain circumstances be as important as in the past (Scambler and Scambler 1984). In this regard instrumental support has been associated with geographical proximity while emotional support, it seems, can be given at a distance (Pearson *et al.* 1993). In terms of gender, women are more likely to facilitate access to professional care and exercise greater control over network members' health behaviours than men,[7] have larger, more multifaceted networks, and report more supportive relationships[8] (e.g. Cornwell 1984; Graham 1987; Shye *et al*. 1995). With regards to *social class*, women from manual working-class families have reported a narrower range of sources of support and have relied more heavily on adult children than women from non-manual families, for whom non-kin and husbands played a more important supportive role (Finlayson 1976).

Most of the literature refers to the positive effect on health status or help seeking of lay networks. However, there is also evidence of detrimental effects. Not all intimate relationships are protective or buffering against the need to use health services (Brown *et al*. 1972; Riessman *et al*. 1991). For example, in one study of intimate relationships for adolescent women who were romantically involved, these relationships were found to have a deterimental effect on health in terms of the reporting of more physical symptoms, and have motivated help seeking. Moreover, it has been found that help seeking which is initiated alone can, in some circumstances, be more effective and appropriate than when significant others are involved (Bleeker *et al*. 1995).

It has been suggested that members of social networks can affect help seeking in a number of ways (Gourash 1978; McKinlay 1972). It is thought that social networks not only buffer the experience of stress which reduces the need for help,[9] but they may also provide emotional support, material aid, services and information, so precluding the necessity for professional assistance. Social networks also transmit norms and values about help seeking. Most important for our analysis here is the way in which social networks act as screening and referral agents to professional services. The involvement of other people is implicated at the point at which contact with formal services is made,[10] and to an extent, social network involvement affects the type of pathway to care. Social networks appear to impact on decision making along a continuum of involvement. Lay people become involved in the decision-making process in a number of ways, depending on the circumstances, symptoms and connectedness of the people involved. The way in which people external to the individual evaluate symptoms, and the point at which they do so, are important in decisions to contact services.[11] The type of behaviour or symptoms exhibited by the person seeking help are also important cues to lay others undertaking the evaluation of symptoms. Anxiety, fear and concern for others have been found to be motivators in lay referral behaviour (Rogers 1990; Roberts 1992; Cornford *et al.* 1993).[12]

Notwithstanding the evidence of the importance of lay networks in help seeking for care, the extent to which lay involvement is important or beneficial in help seeking is a moot point. Reviewed overall, research findings about the importance of social networks in relation to service use have been inconsistent and differ according to condition, type of health action and population group under consideration.[13] There are also suggestions that social networks are not good predictors of health services utilization, or are only of significance in combination with other factors. For example, in one recent study, psychological symptoms and gender were shown to be more relevant predictors of help-seeking behaviour than social networks (Rickwood and Braithwaite 1994),[14] and the findings of a study by Berkanovic and Telesky (1981) suggested that at times lay networks are insignificant or of secondary importance to an individual's own assessment of the need to consult. Contradictory findings are also notable in the literature. For example, in the mental health field, Kadushin (1966) describes how social networks increase the propensity to resort to formal treatment while Suchman (1964) suggests that networks compensate for formal service use. The complicated and contradictory findings of network research suggest that their impact on health utilization and the provision of social support is best assessed by investigating what kinds of people are involved in what networks, with references to situations at various points in the life course and different illness experiences (Estroff and Zimmer 1994).

THE NATURE OF THE INVOLVEMENT OF LAY OTHERS IN HELP SEEKING FOR PRIMARY CARE

The 'Pathways to Care' study provided some examples of the ways in which people were involved and influential in help seeking for contemporary primary care. Three themes are considered here:

1 Advice giving as part of help seeking.
2 The nature of the relationship between people and decisions to seek care.
3 Proxy consultations and the rationing of the use of services.

Advice giving as part of help seeking

Advice giving and lay care can delay or exacerbate a decision to contact formal services. About two-thirds of those interviewed said that during the episodes of illness reported in the diaries their friends or relatives offered advice about self-care or about some form of treatment.[15]

The impact of lay advice and influence on help seeking varied considerably and depended on the particular circumstances people were in. Advice may be proffered or requested, acted upon or ignored. Advice giving differed according to type of symptom and the relationship that existed between people in different contexts. People helped their relatives or friends by describing the way in which *they* had been treated for similar illness or they suggested certain foods or medicines that could be bought with or without a prescription. Relatives offered books or magazines about self care and practical help with lifting when necessary. Friends offered to cook for people when they were ill or take messages or do washing or provide transport. Many people included in this sample reported that they had parents, brothers or sisters living in the same area. Some people said that they had daily contact with one or other of these close relatives. One young woman, for example, said that she asked her mother for advice on health matters most days, and in return she reminded her mother to take her many pills. One couple, a man aged 47 and his wife aged 48, described how they relied on friends and their parents when sick. A third of the interviews were carried out on a large council estate. While many of the respondents living on the estate described close family and friendship ties, one woman pointed out that she could not rely on everyone for support. She said:

> *B is a funny estate. Amongst the older people there's quite a lot of community spirit, and people will help each other out, but a lot of the newer, I would say from the forties and younger, that are on the estate, they couldn't give a damn.*

Work settings were also places where advice was sought and obtained. One respondent, a nurse, described the way in which colleagues tried to help each other. This woman's husband had been ill with 'flu and bronchitis. The interviewer asked her who she turned to for advice. She replied:

> *I usually bounce it off ... there is M, who I work with at the weekend and I usually bounce things off her ... we only see*

each other at work. We have a friend who we work with who has lots of health problems and we try our best to help her, and then it's, it's a little group if you like. You know on Saturday night you are supposed to go off for breaks and we don't, we just sit and natter all night about things.

One woman who worked as a classroom assistant was concerned about her heart. She said she talked to many people about her condition, including the science teacher at school, the school nurse, the physiotherapist and the instructor at the gym. The interviewer asked her about her contacts at school. The woman said that she saw the teacher and the nurse every day, and that she 'mithered' them to death over her heart. This woman also asked her sister to ask her aromatherapy teacher about oils for her children's asthma.

The type and duration of the condition that one is seeking help for is relevant in the provision and acceptance of advice. Where there is a positive relationship with others this can reinforce the propensity towards 'self-help' for an easily identifiable acute condition. This is indicated by the quote below of a woman's account of her reasons for heeding colleagues' health advice in relation to a gastrointestinal problem:

In the pub where I worked, I've known them for years, they were all dead concerned and they all said, 'Have you tried this, have you tried that?', so one said, 'Try arrowroot in a bit of water, mix it up and it soaks it up, bungs it up'. I know it sounds daft but I did come home and try that.

Although potentially stigmatizing and embarrassing, acute physical symptoms seem to lend themselves to identifiable interventions which make advice giving easier than in relation to psychological or personal problems. In the later there may be greater difficulties in the provision and acceptance of, or giving of, appropriate advice. This is indicated in the case of this woman who experienced depression and anxiety following the death of her baby, which propelled her into seeking formal help while no advice was offered or sought from lay others. This outcome seemed to have resulted from a combination of a reluctance to seek advice and the perception of a lack of available emotional support:

Interviewer: Did you have anybody to talk to in terms of friends and family?
Respondent: No, not really my husband, he was very, very

> *upset. But once she was buried and they handed
> the casket over, he sealed the door and that was it.
> He'd put it in its own little box and that was it. He
> didn't want to talk about it. My Mum is 83 so I
> couldn't really go to her and I didn't want to
> burden her. I didn't want to burden anybody . . .
> Everybody at work was sympathetic but I didn't
> want to burden them. I thought, 'Well, everyone
> has enough problems of their own without me
> going pouring it all out to them . . .*

Thus, advice for psychological or personal problems may be less
readily available than advice for other health problems, suggested
by this and previous qualitative research about mental health
(Rogers *et al.* 1976).[16] The scarcity or difficulty of obtaining support and advice may indicate a pattern of help seeking which is
more individualistic than for other conditions[17] and the ability to
articulate and give expression to a psychological or personal problem vis-à-vis problems which are identified as having a physical
cause may also be a relevant factor. Returning to a point made in
Chapter 3, some people do not actively seek help from lay others
or primary care services, e.g. 'I didn't seek help – he (GP) picked
up on it.' The lack of a conscious formulation of need for which
help is sought may also be a reason for the lack of involvement
from lay others.

At times it may be the negative reaction to a person's illness
rather than 'advice' which influences help seeking. One woman
described the incentives to seek help as being the result of the negative reaction of her employer to her illness:

> Interviewer: *Did you mention it to your employer that you had
>   a cough?*
> Respondent: *Well, he knew I was coughing and that and he
>   said, 'Oh have you brought your bugs in?' He said
>   'What have you come in for?'*

The nature of relationships between people and decisions to seek care

The nature of the relationship between the person seeking advice
and others provides some insight into the reasons for diversity in
the way social networks operate as screening and referral agents.
Kinship ties, for example, tend to offer material assistance and

long-term commitments, while friends provide knowledge outside the family group and offer ties based on affection. Thus Salloway and Dillon (1973) speculate that people are more reluctant to rely on friends than family members for continuing support and might therefore contact formal health services more quickly when family support is not available. Lay others, on the other hand, who are not family members, are less likely to tolerate delay in help seeking due to normalization or denial of symptoms (Salloway and Dillon 1973; Alonzo 1980; Calnan 1983).[18]

In the 'Pathways to Care' study, the way in which people came to a decision depended to a large extent on their living and domestic arrangements. Thus, those who were living on their own had, by definition, little choice other than to rely on their own resources and decisions. In fact, the experience of living with an illness, for some, seemed to lead to greater self-possession about the decision to seek help and greater confidence gained through the experience of managing illness over time. This is indicated by this man in his sixties who had been experiencing angina for a number of years:

> *I mean the situation is that with the complaint that I've got, I feel I need to go in, I'll make an appointment to go in. It's no good wasting their time if you're not suffering.*

Having experienced angina for a long time, this man considered himself knowledgeable about the issue. He therefore felt himself to be in a position to advise others, but not to receive advice from others himself:

> *Respondent: If you know they've got angina [other people], you ask, 'What medications are you taking?', and if they say they are on, that beta blocker, I say, 'How does it affect you?', and after they've told me, I'll say, 'You want to come off that.'*
> *Interviewer: So do they ever give you advice?*
> *Respondent: Well no, they are only just starting on that road aren't they?*

Some retired couples, or those who spent a lot of time together, tended to go in for joint decision making. The career point of an illness was also relevant. An important message from people's accounts about the negotiation of seeking help for primary care is the myriad of styles of negotiation, covert conflict and power dynamics. Interpersonal relationships were bound up with different elements of power which appeared to influence the ways in which contact with services were made. At times it was evident that decision making between two individuals was mutual and negotiated. In the first example below, the man and his partner have different but in-depth knowledge about the condition from which she is suffering. He has been deaf for many years and she was a Registered General Nurse. In the second example a woman assumed the authority to call out the out-of-hours doctor without any apparent negotiation with her husband:

> Respondent: *Errm, yeah I had pain all down the side of my face one day and the next day I blew my nose and I went dizzy and my ear popped, so I thought that's what it is.*
> Interviewer: *Right. Did you talk to your husband about it?*
> Respondent: *Oh yeah.*
> Interviewer: *So who knows more about ear infections, your husband or you?*
> Respondent: *I don't know really (laughs), probably quite equal.*
> Interviewer: *Did you both come to the conclusion that it was a middle ear infection?*
> Respondent: *Yeah between the two of us.*
> Interviewer: *What did you decide to do next?*
> Respondent (wife): *I just phoned the doctor.*
> Respondent (husband): *Well I didn't call the doctor, my wife called the doctor unknown to me, or else I wouldn't have been getting him in.*

This man's wife also took on the role of negotiating with the doctor in terms of assessing the severity of pain and the need for the doctor to attend:

> *When my wife rang he said, 'Is it necessary for us to come out?' and I think she thought it was because the pain was really severe.*

Rather than a one-off or superficial piece of advice, involvement of lay others can involve a degree of persistence and tenaciousness which can take place over a considerable period of time. This temporalizing dimension was most notable in couples who spent a lot of time together, either through unemployment or retirement. For example, one man who had 'normalized' the swelling in his groins for eight years, putting it down to the 'ageing process', accounted for his visit to primary care with reference to his wife's involvement:

Interviewer: *So if you put a time on from when you first noticed*
               any swelling to when you'd gone to the doctor,
               how long has that been?
Respondent: *I had the swelling for years, it might have been*
               eight years or more. But from like when the wife
               said to be going that's the last six months. The wife
               kept on saying, 'Go in and see what it is, it's got to
               be something, that', and I thought, Oh it's some-
               thing that happens to everybody at old age and
               what have you, creeping up on you, something to
               do with that. But I went.

The fact that the swelling was not considered to be serious and
there was no pain meant that in this case it was the wife's persistence rather than the husband's medical state which led to referral
to the GP and subsequently to referral to the secondary care
sector.

Proxy consultations and the rationing of the use of services

Proxy consultations are at the extreme end of the continuum of the
way in which others are involved in seeking help from primary care,
and are common in primary care.[19] One of the most common situations in which one person is involved in help seeking from primary
care for another is that of mothers acting as 'proxies' for their
young children. Access to prescribed drugs such as antibiotics,
which are only available from a practising medical practitioner, has
been found to be one of the reasons for consultation (Cornford *et
al.* 1993), and as we saw in the last chapter, mothers evaluate children's illness behaviour according to subtle behavioural cues
judged against their children's 'normal' behaviour.

Accounts from mothers in our study suggested that in seeking
help from primary care services mothers' own needs for services
were relegated in importance to their children's. There were nine
families in the qualitative sample that had two or three children
under nine years of age. Of these families three mothers said that
they did not have time to look after their own health. This resulted
in self-rationing of primary care services. Accounts included comments on the need not to 'mither' the doctor, choosing the pharmacist to treat their own illnesses, and 'saving' visits to the GP for
when their children were sick. One mother, when asked why she

continued to use a doctor with whom she was dissatisfied, said that because she used the 'good' doctor at the practice for both of her children who were frequently sick, she did not feel able to use this doctor for herself as well. Instead she 'made do' with the less competent doctor who was also more available given his perceived lack of popularity among patients on the health centre's list. Mothers' rationing of health care for themselves seemed to add legitimacy to requests for primary care help for their children:

> *I've put off calling the doctor for myself. If it's for me, I'd rather wait.*

> *I don't like calling the doctor in the middle of the night. I called in the morning. I try not to get him to come to me, I'd rather go to them. If I think it's relatively serious myself, I would more or less demand the doctor see the child.*

Another young woman was busy looking after two boys, both under two years of age. She told the interviewer that she had had a lot of trouble with her back and ought to return to the physiotherapist once a fortnight, but could only 'grin and bear it'. When asked why she was not attending for treatment she replied:

> *Because I haven't got time. Too busy dealing with my kids and everything else to bother about myself. I work weekend nights, and when I've sorted the kids out, I don't really bother about myself. I could be crippled and not even bother then.*

Another mother had a similar story. She had to care for three young children. She said that she suffered agony with arthritis in her neck, but could not go to the physiotherapist because she could not leave the children with anyone and she did not like to leave her baby. Her mother-in-law suggested lavender baths, but she explained why she did not follow her advice:

> *It sounds nice, I just don't get round to doing it. It's just time, and it's different with kiddies.*

Mothers' decision making about their children related to their claims about knowing their children intimately and best. This may exclude others, who are not seen as having the same type of knowledge, from the decision-making process. One woman when asked whether her husband (who was unemployed and at home all the time) had been consulted about the decision responded:

*No I just know, I know myself when my kids, when there is
something wrong.*

This assumed authority as a proxy extended beyond mothers'
making decisions about sick young children since women frequently acted as proxies on behalf of other members of the family.

Those caring for elderly or sick people may also find that their
caring role makes it difficult for them to seek help when sick themselves. Four people discussed their roles as full-time carers, and
three said that they did not have time to look after their own health.
One woman was caring for her 59-year-old husband. He was seriously ill, waiting for a heart bypass operation. His wife suffered
from high blood pressure and depression, but she told the interviewer:

I don't have time to be sick, that's the problem.

Later in the interview she said that if she was ill with a cold herself
she took 'hot toddies', but had to 'carry on'. Another elderly
woman was caring for her husband. He was seriously ill, having had
a stroke. The eye specialist had told this woman that she should
have her blood pressure checked. One day she had to see the GP to
discuss her husband's poor health, so while she was at the surgery
she took the opportunity to ask about her own blood pressure. It
was slightly raised and she was told to return to the health centre in
a month for another check-up. However, she told the interviewer:

*Well, there was no way I could go back, L [her husband] was
getting more and more difficult. And so I've never been back,
you see, and it just sort of ticked around in the back of my mind
that one day this had got to be done.*

SUMMARY

The data presented from our study on the patterns of help seeking
show the variety of pathways to the doctor. The latter involve
different timescales, action and contact with people. Some of the
similarities and variations in patterns of help seeking can be
accounted for by the type of illness experienced by individuals.
However, it is likely that other differences cannot be explained
mainly by reference to the nature of the illness alone. People's ability to contain illness and the ways in which they do so are interlinked with their situational contexts. In our own study the

undertaking of paid and unpaid work was used to illustrate the ways in which aspects of people's everyday lives can promote or inhibit the effectiveness of coping strategies. Our survey showed that only a small proportion of contacts with primary care were not preceded by attempts to ameliorate illness through self-care and that people who were ill were far more likely to use self-care than professional health services. In the instances where people reported consulting primary care services, the data suggest that people tend to wait some time before resorting to formal primary care services. Moreover when people do use professional care this tends to be in addition to self-care practices. While our quantitative data show that only a small proportion of people were consulted for advice immediately prior to contacting formal primary care, the qualitative data suggested that this is likely to be an underestimate of the ways in which other people are involved in decisions about help seeking. In providing in-depth accounts of illness management and help seeking more generally, people identified an array of the ways in which others were involved.

The qualitative accounts of individuals pointed to the complexities involved in people's help-seeking activities and the influence of other people over a longer timescale rather than discrete episodes of illness for which help is being sought. The involvement of lay others may not be immediate. Lay knowledge about illness and health action is developed over time and 'stored' up for use when needed. Knowledge about a child's health may be gleaned from recent events (e.g. the action and common-sense knowledge gained from an 'epidemic' of 'flu or asthma) and from more ingrained ways of dealing with problems in the family and from other people over a longer period of time. The ways in which people engage with one another and different styles in negotiating the process of help seeking also point to the limitations of viewing help seeking in individualistic terms and confirm the complexities that are involved in interactions about health within households. Finally, there was also evidence of mothers and carers relegating their own needs and rationing the use of health services for themselves as a way of ensuring that appropriate treatment is gained for their children and others. There were suggestions too of a gendered pattern of help seeking in which women acted as proxies for men who did not wish to articulate their health needs, and where contact with formal health services would not otherwise have occurred. The extensive literature on social networks points to the way in which other people are sometimes a medium for the exchange of ideas, advice and information about help seeking.

This is also important in considering the provision of informal care which is examined in the next chapter. The provision of lay primary care may circumvent the need to use services or provide an additional source of care alongside that provided by formal primary care services. Other mediators of demand are also implicated in influencing patterns of demand and help seeking. In Chapter 7 we examine how pharmacists play an important role as mediators between social networks and health professionals, as providers of primary care and as a resource for self-care.

NOTES

1 It should be noted that the purpose of any feasibility study is to test procedures and methods and it is therefore not possible to guarantee precise results. We are currently in the process of validating the data and any known inaccuracies are addressed in the text when appropriate. It should also be remembered that the sample size of the feasibility study is relatively small. Some of the analyses are based on very small numbers and the results should be treated with caution.

2 See the Appendix for further details about the design and content of the feasibility study.

3 Contact with formal primary care services is defined as contact with a GP, practice nurse, or a doctor or nurse from an Accident and Emergency Department. Also included are contacts with pharmacists where the respondent asked the pharmacist for advice.

4 The overall fit of the model is not very good: a likelihood ratio Chi square of 42.3 with 14 degrees of freedom. This is caused by highly dispersed data. Although there are tests and techniques to deal with dispersed data, this was not considered necessary. The analysis is exploratory and the results are presented for illustrative purposes only.

5 In relation to help seeking more specifically, professionals working outside the health service may also be of importance temporarily. These groups constitute the clergy, social workers, police officers and employers, teachers or lay strangers, such as passers-by or shop-owners (Calnan 1983). These people might bring into decision making official health knowledge (the police, for example, receive formal first aid training), as well as operating with lay constructs of health and illness (Rogers 1990). In terms of help seeking for services, involvement in decisions about other people's health is likely to be influenced by the moral obligation and legal implications associated with those who have a formally ascribed public or professional role, which implicates lower thresholds of perception of the need for medical attention because of moral, social and legal pressures.

6 The 1994 Health and Life Styles survey found that in terms of feeling socially supported, talking to friends, relatives and neighbours on the phone was more common than visiting friends.

7 Although they are more likely than men to be more critical of the level and quality of support.

8 Despite this evidence, the focus on women (as opposed to gender in recent research) has in comparative terms left the role of men and the interactive character of family and health networks and participation of family members underexamined (Prout 1988; Miles 1991; Backett 1992). There is, for example, some evidence to suggest that social networks work differently for women than for men (Verbrugge 1985) and there are alternative ways of understanding men's health behaviour.

9 Aspects of caring and nurturance and a close confiding relationship have a protective function, and recent research suggests that social support from kin and friends is important for counteracting stressful events which might otherwise lead to formal help seeking, including from primary care services (Kadushin 1966; Oakley 1992; Pini *et al.* 1995; Reif *et al.* 1995).

10 For instance, the prompt seeking of help for acute myocardial infarction has been associated with the presence of a supportive social network (Bleeker *et al.* 1995) and those entering psychotherapy have generally been found to be well connected in their social systems, with numerous strong ties, close friends, romantic relationships and confidantes (Bankoff 1994).

11 Alonzo (1984) examined the impact of the family on care seeking during a suspected episode of acute coronary artery disease. The advice of family and lay others significantly affected physician consultation but it did so in different ways according to the type of symptoms being presented by the individual and the closeness of interpersonal relationships. When individuals were found to be experiencing 'prodromal symptoms' (the type of symptoms which precede the onset of acute signs and symptoms in myocardial infarction), assistance from spouses resulted in a greater likelihood of physician consultation than when lay others were not involved. However, during the acute phase informing a spouse of severe symptoms did not always lead to expeditious care seeking. Individuals who initially informed their spouses experienced a significantly longer delay in contacting services, whereas informing non-family others shortened the lay evaluation phase. Men were much more likely to lengthen the 'lay evaluation phase' when consulting female partners than vice versa.

12 Research has shown, for example, that there is a greater likelihood of lay advisers calling the police where threat to others is perceived than when it isn't (Rogers 1990). A study of the beliefs and evaluations of children's illness among a group of mothers who had consulted a general practitioner because of a cough found that a major concern for

mothers was their fear that their child was going to die (Cornford *et al.* 1993). In a study of professionals' and parents' perception of A and E use in a children's hospital the decision to use the hospital rather than the GP was at times related by mothers themselves to their own degree of anxiety (Roberts 1992).

13 Berkanovic and Telesky (1981), using a multiple regression analysis, estimated that 57 per cent of the variance in decisions to seek medical care was related directly to symptoms while 41 per cent was explained by symptom-specific network advice and beliefs. Suchman (1964) estimated that three out of four people consult lay people before attending a doctor's surgery. Calnan (1983) reported 81 per cent of a large sample of GP attenders having had contact with at least one person in a decision-making process related to A and E attendance. Patients who had contact with more than one person constituted only 2 per cent of the overall sample.

14 For example, in a study of social psychological factors affecting help seeking for emotional problems, psychological symptoms and gender were shown to be more relevant predictors of help-seeking behaviour than social network, and social support was found to be important in general help seeking but not for those with evident emotional distress (Rickwood and Braithwaite 1994).

15 Aspects of this are looked at in more detail in the next chapter.

16 Although when such advice and support is forthcoming it seems to be viewed and valued positively by people.

17 This is currently being examined in a project on the management of depression within primary care.

18 Calnan found that when neighbours or friends were the contacts the decision to seek medical care was made within three hours in 81 per cent of the cases, compared with only 67 per cent when relatives were the contacts. On the basis of these findings Calnan argued that 'neighbours and friends, when put in the position of adviser, may tend to be more cautious because of the moral responsibility of taking risks with other people's health or other people's children (1983: 27).

19 An analysis of 12,499 out-of-hours calls found that 50 per cent of the callers were requesting help for themselves, while the remainder made the call for another family member, usually a child. Most individuals who called were found to have discussed the problem with family or friends before calling.

6

SELF- AND LAY-CARE IN MANAGING ILLNESS

The basic premise of self care is that individuals have the ability to influence their health and to participate in their health care. Self care is defined ... as those activities initiated or performed by an individual, family or community to achieve, maintain or promote maximum health potential.

(Steiger and Lipson)

There can be little doubt that self-care practices are pervasive, and a 'normal' response to everyday symptoms and problems of health and illness ... Furthermore, self-care represents a common way in which most people attempt to prevent illness and disability and one of the principal ways in which positive health behaviour is generally promoted.

(De Friese *et al.*, *Social Science and Medicine*)

INTRODUCTION

As we saw in the last chapter, everyday help seeking for primary care, self-care and informal care are intrinsically bound up with one another. This chapter is concerned with examining in greater depth the lay management of illness. In this regard the focus of analysis moves away from patients as *recipients* of professional services to ways in which people act as *providers* of primary care. In its narrowest sense, self-care is associated with the range of diagnostic, curative and rehabilitative action that people undertake themselves to preserve health or manage illness (Shuval *et al.* 1989). Self-care can be a supplement to professional care or it may occur separately. Self-care activities have attracted attention from those wishing to understand wider social and cultural influences on health. In this broader sense, self-care has been linked to the subjective identities of population groups, active self-monitoring and the conscious adoption of healthy lifestyles. Self-help, which is imbued with a philosophy of holism, has been described as drawing together the fragmented experience of health and illness (i.e. psychological, physical and social strands) which act to reinforce the wholeness of personal relationships (May 1997).

This chapter is mainly concerned with examining self-care in the narrower sense noted above. It focuses in particular on the role of self-care as a form of primary care, outside the formal health care sector. However, at times, the wider social significance of self-care as a distinctive lifestyle and form of consumption is relevant to an understanding of our motives and actions in undertaking self-care activities and use of services. In the final section of the chapter the contribution of lay others and self-help groups to providing care outside formal primary care are considered. We will also look at the interface between lay and professional approaches to self-care. Sources of information about self-care and alternatives are also important. This topic will be discussed in the next chapter.

SELF-CARE IN THE POLICY CONTEXT OF DEMAND MANAGEMENT

The interest in promoting self-care practices has diverse roots. A 'bottom-up' self-care movement has gained considerable momentum over the last two decades (Anderson *et al.* 1991). New social movements dissatisfied with the practices of health care delivery (particularly in relation to women's health, physical disability and mental health) have questioned the effectiveness and benefits of contact with health services. Within these new social movements, self-care has been one aspect of individuals' taking more control over their own health independent of, in spite of, or even in opposition to, professional care. The promotion of self-care has also come 'top-down' from the State and in recent years has become part of official health care policy across different health care systems. For example, in the US, self-care and self-help are viewed as parts of managed health care systems.

Self-care has a potentially important role to play in determining patterns of demand and use of primary care. Although the potential of self-care to reduce health expenditure has, according to some, been exaggerated, increased self-care may act to reduce or contain the use of services. It may also transfer activities from the formal to the informal health care sector. Self-medication, for example, has been a means of shifting some costs of health care from the state to consumers (Blenkinsop and Bradley 1996). International trends towards deregulation of prescription-only to pharmacy medicines have increased the potential for lay choice in symptom treatment. Similarly, the reduction in eligibility for free prescriptions in the UK means that fewer individuals have a financial incentive to seek treatment from a doctor. Consequently they are more likely to go directly to a pharmacist and miss out the surgery. Changes in community and continuing care services have also placed greater emphasis on the care of dependent people in their own homes and neighbourhoods. This involves a greater reliance on the lay management of care. The growing popularity of the World Wide Web offers new opportunities for the development and promotion of self-care activities. 'On line' patient meetings for illnesses such as diabetes and cancer together with Internet health information sites provide the bases for a global source of health and social support which can be accessed by ordinary people (Feenberg *et al*. 1996).

Despite these trends, there is considerable uncertainty about the extent to which self-care acts as an *alternative* to or *supplement* to formally provided primary care. The use of home pregnancy tests and other home testing technology (e.g. electronic blood pressure monitors, cholesterol testers and blood sugar monitors) are examples of products made available directly to the public via community pharmacies. However, what remains ambiguous is the extent to which direct access reduces, rather than duplicates, these tests routinely available from primary care. How do primary care professionals respond to self-testing? How frequently are pregnancy tests quickly replicated in a formal primary care setting for validation? These pertinent questions still await answers.

The framing of self-care is a factor in the way in which it is taken into account in the planning and delivery of health care services. To date, the trend towards lay management of illness has been met with both enthusiasm and caution. It has been depicted as both empowering for individuals and excessively individualistic and victim blaming. Anderson *et al*. (1991: 102), for example, claim that 'illness management is often reduced to individual capabilities, divorcing the personal from the complex socio-political, cultural and economic context'. The point has also been made that a focus on lifestyle and the benefits of lay care cannot substitute for addressing structural and environmental factors which produce disease and that self-care is infrequently placed in this light (Dean 1986). This points to the need to view self-care practices within a framework which takes into account issues of equity and context. One means of understanding both the potential and limitations of self-care practices is to examine what people actually do in the way of self-care and the values and meanings they attribute to these activities. Thus, in this next section, we turn to exploring the meaning and nature of self-care practices and their relationship to service utilization.

SELF-CARE PRACTICES

Self-care covers a wide set of activities ranging from adoption of particular lifestyles to illness reduction strategies. One set of self-care activities is not necessarily predictive of others. Barofsky (1978) distinguishes between four types of self-care behaviour:

1 regulatory self-care (e.g. personal hygiene, sleeping),
2 preventative self-care (e.g. exercise, dieting),
3 reactive self-care (self-treatment as a response to symptoms),
4 restorative self-care, compliance with personal care and treatment.

In this chapter we are mainly concerned with the third type.

Individual self-care is one option among many when experiencing symptoms. People tend to do what is pragmatic based on what they perceive will work. For example, they may choose multiple treatments which may mix conventional and alternative approaches. As Eyles and Donovan (1990: 78) point out: 'coping with illness takes many forms and can encompass several different attempts to deal with one particular condition'. Dean (1986) has suggested four alternative forms of illness behaviour once symptoms have been recognized:

1 decisions to do nothing about symptoms,
2 self-medication,
3 non-medication forms of self-treatment,
4 decisions to consult professional providers.

The last of these has been dealt with in a previous chapter. The emphasis here is on the first three of these behaviours.

Non-action about symptoms

In comparison to the other three areas of illness behaviour, relatively little is known about the extent to which people decide to do nothing about identified illness. This is partly as a result of interpreting the meaning and ambiguities of non-action as an illness management strategy. The notion of non-action has two aspects: literal non-action (i.e. the sufferer does nothing at all about his or her symptoms), and avoidance of service utilization. Estimates of these vary according to the type of experienced illness. The meaning of doing nothing is also morally ambiguous. It could denote either an unwise neglect of symptoms that should and could be responded to, or a wise illness-management strategy. (Judgements about these two might only be possible retrospectively.)

Non-action in relation to the presence of symptoms has been interpreted in a variety of ways. Implicit to many of the traditional 'clinical iceberg' studies is the assumption that untreated symptoms represent unmet need. Terms such as 'delay in seeking medical attention' and 'late presentation'[1] also imply that non-action is undesirable. The failure to obtain treatment for untreated symptoms has been attributed to negative psychological traits on the part of individuals and to a means of personal control and coping.[2] Moreover, as we discussed in Chapter 4, the presence of symptoms is often regarded as a normal part of everyday life and good health. Though it is rarely considered in epidemiological research, 'no treatment' action can be a means of effective management. Eyles and Donovan (1990) found that non-action is at times viewed as a 'means of coping' and was often seen as the first strategy to adopt in relation to the onset of an illness. The importance of being able to cope on one's own is a reason for opting for a non-action strategy. For example, in relation to mental health, a recent study found that the need for privacy and the threat of disclosure were reasons for self-reliance and non-action in relation to the experience of personal and emotional troubles. In particular, a personal disclosure was viewed as risking a loss of face which might add to, rather than mitigate, existing difficulties (Rogers *et al.* 1997a). The risk of loss may relate to material and social resources, for example in relation to gaining life insurance coverage for a number of conditions.

In a study of mothers' responses to their children's illnesses, Cunningham-Burley and Irvine (1987) found that the most common symptoms for which no action was taken were respiratory symptoms, changes in behaviour, such as tiredness or irritability, followed by sickness and diarrhoea, rashes and spots. In a Danish study which examined behavioural responses to common symptoms, the percentage of people taking non-action ranged from 7 per cent of the respondents who had influenza to 29 per cent who did nothing about chest pains. A follow-up study after a six-month interval found that 37 per cent of the conditions had not been treated in any way and that non-action related to both acute-temporary and longer term conditions (Dean 1986).

In Chapter 4 it was noted that people often learned the limitations of services. This was sometimes reinforced by the fatalism of contact with health professionals, who may attempt to normalize illness in an attempt to reassure patients. A fatalistic acceptance of a condition was also a reason for taking no action, which was evident in the accounts of some of the individuals interviewed in the 'Pathways to Care' study. The following man, for example, took no action for the swelling in his groin and commented:

> *I thought it's something that happens to everybody at old age and what have you, creeping up on you.*

Similarly, a man suffering regularly from back pain brought on by lifting awkwardly came to expect back pain when lifting. He accommodated to his symptoms because he had an understanding of their source in everyday activities:

> *Oh no, these things happen and I just considered them to take a normal course. At the back of my mind when it happened I've thought well, three or four days and it will ease off and I'll be back at work and that's basically the way it happened.*

The illness trajectory is also important in so far as people take no action for common and easily identifiable problems but may change the strategy when the perception of what is wrong also changes. One of the women, for example, was happy to do nothing about her pain until her view about her problem changed and she chose to consult the GP instead:

> *The pain I thought maybe it was because I'd been sitting in a draught. I thought it may be a touch of neuralgia, but then in the morning when I got up it was obvious it was this ear thing.*

While at times no action could be seen among our respondents as a form of radical non-intervention, at other times reasons for non-action or taking up alternative action was a result of deference to medical authority and to formal medical care. This is discussed in more detail in the final section of this chapter.

Self-medication

There are three types of self-medication which are under the direct control of the lay individual:

- the use of substances considered to maintain health or prevent illness,
- the treatment of self-limiting conditions or early stages of more serious illness,
- treatment taken in addition to professionally prescribed medication.

Self-medication is recognized as being widely prevalent. Recently, Blenkinsop and Bradley (1996) have noted that sales of non-prescribed or 'over the counter' (OTC) medicines in 1994 were the equivalent of one-third of the NHS drug bill. In any two-week period, nine out of ten people will experience symptoms and there is evidence that OTC medicine is used to treat one in four symptoms. Increases in consumption of OTC medicine are likely to be a result of a combination of changes in demand and supply factors. These include the lowering of normative thresholds at which sickness absence is justified and treatment considered appropriate (Dunnell and Cartwright 1972), and the deregulation of some medicines previously only available on prescription. Self-medication practices are also likely to be shaped by advertising, the financial resources of individuals (Mitra *et al.* 1993) and communication within and between social networks (Dunnell and Cartwright 1972).

Self-medication is frequently the first active response to treating an episode of illness. Cunningham-Burley and Irvine (1987) note in a study of the lay management of children's illnesses that buying analgesics and bottles of cough medicine were the most common responses to symptoms. In our 'Pathways to Care' study, prospective data from health diaries showed that the most common response to illness was the taking of OTC medication (80 per cent of those reporting restricted activity over the 4 weeks took OTC medicines). Homeopathic and herbal medications are also an increasing source of self-medication for both chronic and acute illnesses. Estimates of OTC purchases of herbal and homeopathic remedies suggest that this form of home remedy has increased at a rate of 15–20 per cent every year over the last five years. It is worth more than £18 million at the level of 1995 retail prices (personal communication with Welleda).

There appears to be a degree of ambivalence from official health sources about the risks and benefits of self-medication practices and at times a preoccupation with the appropriateness and the regulation of self-medication. For example, a Norwegian study which examined the lay management and self-medication of fever reported that one-fifth of the sample undertook 'inappropriate measuring of body temperature'. The authors argue on the basis of their results that there is 'a need for more definite and consistent information to make fever management and self medication more rational'. Implicit in this line of argument are assumptions that self-medication is fundamentally different from taking prescribed medication and that all medication should ultimately be managed by health care personnel. However, the dichotomy between the use of self-obtained and medically prescribed drugs may have been over-drawn. For example, in a recent Italian study, Calva (1996) found that while medication and drug purchases of antibiotics without medical prescriptions were common, the majority of antibiotics were in fact prescribed by a physician. The misuse of antibiotics was relevant to those who had obtained them either *with* or *without* a physician prescription, suggesting the need for appropriate 'education' of both professionals and patients. Similarly, before they were superseded by less toxic drugs, the old tricyclic antidepressants accounted for one-third of all suicides. Arguably then, in practice, no neat line exists between prescribed medication (implicitly safe/ proper) and self-medication (implicitly unsafe/ improper).

The meaning attached to self-medication practices by those undertaking them is to an extent likely to be different from an official medical viewpoint. The reasons lay people give for self-medication practices suggest that control over the therapeutic process and self-knowledge may be more important than perceived efficacy. Compared to 'official' views, differences in lay perspectives on the meanings attached to medication practices and on the effect of drugs are highlighted by research which shows that illicit or harmful drugs have been used by people for therapeutic effects. For example, alcohol ingestion has been found to be used for the relief of anxiety symptoms and cocaine for relief of symptoms associated with attention-deficit hyperactivity disorder (Horner *et al.* 1996). Similarly, smoking and illicit drugs have been used as a form of self-medication for anxiety and depression (Lerman *et al.* 1996). Eyles and Donovan (1990) found that among their sample of lay respondents, smoking was viewed as important for alleviating stress and chesty symptoms. It was also reported to have a soothing, calming effect which helped to counterbalance worries which are perceived to cause serious conditions. Similarly, some people use smoking as a means of maintaining positive mental health (Rogers *et al.* 1997b). A study of substance use among male street prostitutes found a direct link between substance use and economic dependence on prostitution (Morse *et al.* 1992). People also appear to use self- and prescribed medication in response to situations which arise as part of everyday life rather than as distinct categories of drugs, in the same way health professionals do for circumscribed use. For example, there is some evidence that the retention of prescribed drugs for future use is a common practice. In a study of self-treatment prior to consultation in a Danish general practice, it was found that a large amount of medicine used for self-treatment was prescription medicine stored from an earlier time (Dean 1986). Additionally for the treatment of minor ailments, cost and convenience are at times more relevant in decisions to self-medicate (versus obtaining prescribed medication) than substantive differences in the nature of the product or the medical advice which accompanies the latter (Schafheutle *et al.* 1996).

Home remedies and non-medication self-treatment

Home remedies are often used to treat conditions 'not worthy of a doctor', where traditional treatment is considered to have failed or to be ineffective, or to avoid the side effects of traditional regimens (Thorogood 1990). While most of the literature suggests that self-treatments are directed at the reduction of symptoms, there is some evidence that preventing symptoms or protective responses are also a focus of non-medication self-care activities. The use of home remedies is sometimes seen as a continuation of self-medication practices. At other times they receive separate consideration. Dean (1986), for example, treats home remedies as distinct from self-medication, conceptualizing them as a synthesis of learning and experience. Cunningham-Burley and Irvine (1987) found that many of the home nursing responses adopted by mothers in relation to their children were modelled on standard medical advice (e.g. the use of tepid sponging in relation to fever reduction).

A number of studies illustrate the considerable range of non-medication activities used by lay people in response to illness, including alteration of diets; the taking of or changing of exercise regimen; rest; having a holiday; reducing workload; taking fresh air; bed rest; poultices; and the use of appliances such as heat pads. Home remedies include rest, rubbing, gargling, bandaging and other 'simple procedures'. Cunningham-Burley and Irvine (1987) found that home nursing care (such as dealing with cuts and grazes, providing drinks, encouraging a child to rest and eat) was a common response to symptoms and children's illness behaviour.

Responses are of course also condition-specific. Increasing fluid intake and rest are frequently reported responses to influenza and colds. Avoiding lifting or stooping, and the use of heat pads, massage, increased rest and exercise have been found to be common responses to lumbar pain. Chest pain is treated by a reduction in the pace of activities and by reducing smoking (Dean 1986).

Estimates of the level of use of home remedies vary significantly. Low estimates of prevalence may be due to health care professionals, researchers and other commentators viewing such activities as marginal or irrelevant compared to mainstream health care practices.[3] Limiting the definition of self-treatment to home appliances, herbal medications and various forms of home remedies is a way of approximating self-care to the traditional health care responses which might exclude other beneficial forms of self-care. Dean (1986) widens the notion of non-medication self-care to include 'coping behaviour' in the general management of stress. Freer (1980) included a category of 'social medical' activities, such as spending time with the family or friends and going out for lunch in his definition of self-care. Sickness absence, while traditionally viewed as a *need* variable in health services research, can also be seen as a form of self-care since it involves the person staying at home and reducing normal activities. It could also be warranted as a preventative activity at times when isolating infection from work colleagues. Religious beliefs have been found to be a source of solace and strength. Religious beliefs were found to provide ways of coping and recovering through faith in God (Eyles and Donovan 1990).

Some research show lifestyle differences between social groups, with self-care practices being generationally and culturally linked. A Danish self-care study found that skilled workers and salaried employees remained in bed during periods of illness, while self-employed business people, housewives and unskilled workers more often maintained normal routines. Younger people were more likely than older people to respond to depression by discussing problems with someone in their social network (Dean 1986). Blaxter and Paterson (1982) found the use of home remedies more prevalent among the older generation of Scottish women compared with the younger women who were more likely to use proprietary medicines. The low use of home remedies was also a feature of the reported behaviours of young mothers in the Cunningham-Burley and Irvine (1987) study in the 1980s. Rapid changes in self-care practices may happen over fairly short periods of time. Elliott-Binns (1986), comparing the results of two surveys conducted over a ten-year period between the mid-1970s and mid-80s, notes that home remedies were mentioned less often in the later survey, were less 'exotic', and more likely to include remedies like hot lemon drinks. The use of homeopathic and herbal medicines had grown in popularity, with the highest usage found among the 30–45 year age range.

Different, and a wider range of practices are evident among some ethnic groups. A survey by Jesson *et al.* (1994) found that Afro-Caribbean respondents were more likely than Asian respondents to use traditional remedies, and older respondents were more likely to use them than younger ones. Thirteen per cent of the minority ethnic sample reported having consulted a traditional healer. Afro-Caribbeans were more likely to have consulted an alternative practitioner than Asians a Hakim or Viad. Cultural differences in the use of home remedies have been noted in other studies. Thorogood (1990) found that West Indian women routinely maintain their own and their family's health using 'bush' and home remedies for minor everyday illness. Morgan (1988) found that Afro-Caribbean men's 'non-compliance' with hypertension medication was linked to the use of alternative herbal remedies. These were preferred in order to avoid the perceived negative effects of taking allopathic medication on a long-term basis.

PREDICTORS OF SELF-CARE PRACTICES

Current enthusiasm to view self-care as a regulatory mechanism for demand for formal health care brings with it an interest in identifying which groups in the population already undertake self-care and which individuals might be persuaded to do so. This is currently difficult to ascertain. While some differences between social groups have been noted, the nature of the use of self-care practices appears to be subject to considerable flux and change. Moreover, differences that do exist are equivocal. Empirical results regarding socio-demographic characteristics as correlates of self-care are inconsistent. In quantitative studies there has been a failure to relate health beliefs to particular forms of self-care (Calnan 1989; Greimel *et al.* 1997). Segall and Goldstein (1989) conclude that, overall, no single dimension of self-care can be associated with distinctive social, cultural and economic characteristics. Similarly, at the end of a paper examining the self-care components of lifestyles, while acknowledging that the socio-economic situation exerts a greater influence on self-care behaviours than health attitudes and knowledge, Dean (1989) concludes that socialization and cultural values are major factors which shape people's behaviour.

Some studies have also found a strong relationship between socio-economic status and self-care (Uitenbroek *et al.* 1996). In contrast Dean *et al.* (1983) found weak associations between education, income and self-care responses to common illnesses. However, one clear message from the literature appears to be that access to social resources is a predictor of preference for self-care over formal services (Dean 1989; Greimel *et al.* 1997).

In the pathways to care study the situational and social contexts of illness also impinge on whether and what sort of self-care practice is adopted. As suggested by one young woman from the 'Pathways to Care' study, self-care might sometimes be born out of necessity rather than being an active or positive choice:

> Respondent: *I don't generally go [to the GP] for myself, no. It's mainly my kids. I don't bother with myself, I really don't . . . like if I get the 'flu I just sort it myself.*
> Interviewer: *What do you do?*
> Respondent: *Grin and bear it until it's over.*

She has a large family and her use of self-care rather than the GP seems to be related to her need to manage a complex domestic situation. Demonstrating self-reliance and strength by not using services forms the backdrop to her self-care practices. Efficacy, cost and acceptability were also important factors in making decisions about whether to start and stop self-care practices. For example, one woman reported trying evening primrose oil for arthritis but stopped because she did not get any benefit. Another woman reported very rarely buying OTC medicines because they were deemed by her to be ineffective. A working-class man of 56 who originally took herbal tea for his back pain continued to take it even though it did not alleviate his pain because it made him feel better in himself. Consideration of cost is evident in these two accounts, one from a man and one from a woman with low incomes. First the man:

> Respondent: *I used to have them cod-liver tablets and then I stopped taking them.*

> *Interviewer:*   Have you? Why?
> *Respondent:*   It was just the price of the all ... you know, with
>   being on the social ...
> *Interviewer:*   Are they expensive?
> *Respondent:*   Quite dear, yeah.

The woman, who suffered from chronic and severe headaches, had
wanted to use alternative remedies she had found out about, but
was prevented from doing so because of the cost:

> *Interviewer:*   Have you not thought about any sort of other
>   remedy, like maybe the chemists and asking them,
>   or trying alternative medicine?
> *Respondent:*   Well, actually, it's funny that because I was read-
>   ing that book, you know, all those remedies and
>   herbal things, and it said things you could take
>   for headaches, well you go and price them up in
>   [town], and you need this and that and the other
>   and you think it's going to cost 15 quid for that
>   lot.
> *Interviewer:*   Was that herbal stuff Chinese?
> *Respondent:*   Yeah that's it – but God, when you price it up. We
>   did actually go pricing some of the things up,
>   because they have [town] market and you know
>   the hippies there and they have a lot of herbal
>   things and when we priced it all up, God, I thought
>   it's about 15 quid. I get them every day the
>   headaches, it would cost me about £40 a week for
>   something like that.
> *Interviewer:*   So would you, so basically if they were cheaper
>   would you use them?
> *Respondent:*   Yeah, if they were a lot cheaper I would use
>   them.

In addition to the cost of self-care from some interviews, a deter-
rent to undertaking self-care appeared to be related to who was
seen to have authority in health matters. Some respondents viewed
medical authority as the most appropriate, which in turn is linked to
people's notions of who should have control over medical matters.
This was indicated in this account from a young working class
mother (IE) who reports opting to use the doctor instead of using
self-care or 'modelling' on her mother's actions:

Respondent: My mam has gone to the chemist and bought
things, in a lot of ways I'm like my mam but in a
lot of ways I'm not.
Interviewer: In what ways would you say?
Respondent: Well she'd go to the chemist and she'd get, buy
something, where I wouldn't, I'd go straight to the
problem itself me, I'd rather go to the doctor, than
mess about up here and think, oh God have I got
the right thing, you know, after you've give it them,
you think oh have I done the right thing by him
(the baby) or haven't I?

THE ROLE OF SELF-HELP GROUPS IN
SELF-CARE

Self-care activities involve not only the individual but others in a
person's social network. Inter- and intra-household favours are
often sought and people may ration the circumstances in which they
call for substitute care. Social support is a common form of care
provided to others, which may reinforce, or make possible, people's
own attempts at self-care. Social support refers to emotional,
instrumental and affirmational support, as well as advocacy assistance. These have been related in turn to different combinations of
network provision. Aspects of lay care provided by others which
have direct relevance to self-care are:

- people's perceptions of social support, including the perceived
  availability, as well as the direct effects, of social support which
  have been found to have a direct positive effect on individuals'
  coping strategies,
- the role of social support as a supplement, or alternative to, professional care.

Self-help groups, which have proliferated in the health care arena in
recent years, provide mutual aid, information and support. These
groups have been viewed as providing supplementary sources of
support and care outside people's existing social networks and are a
means of sharing long-term existential problems through emphatic
mutual support. The growth of the Internet has also allowed a new
configuration of 'self-help' groups to emerge. A recent analysis of
the electronic messages logged with a cancer support group of the
Internet showed that the site was used for information giving and

seeking, encouragement and support, expression of personal experience, thanks, humour and prayer (Klemm *et al.* 1998). The proliferation of self-help groups at a time of expansion in formal health care provision suggests that they address problems which are either neglected or inadequately dealt with by professional services. The rise of these groups points to extensive patient responsibility in the context of:

- the failure of existing services to meet self-defined need,
- increasing recognition of the value of mutual help, alongside, or as an alternative to, professional help,
- highlighting self-help and alternative responses to the management of illness.

The benefits of self-help groups for members are undisputed. In terms of goals directed at improving matters for those that participate, self-help groups have been found to be effective in reducing illness-related stress, encouraging feelings of mastery in controlling illness, reducing feelings of isolation, and increasing social activities. Differences have also been reported in changing the opinions of the family and others outside the family, including health professionals. Information gleaned from participating in self-help groups leads to patients representing their interests better when interacting with professionals (Trogan 1989). However, self-care groups cannot, it seems, replace professional services. A survey carried out in the 1980s found that changes in utilization behaviour induced by self-help groups was reported by only 40 per cent of members and that there was an overall *rise* in the use of services. In terms of the health policy implications the authors of the study conclude:

> As our results (in agreement with all other more important studies) show, the outcome of self-help groups hardly overlaps with that of the professional services. Thus the question of whether self-help groups are better or worse than professional services or whether they can replace them is pointless, except in isolated cases. This means that cuts in social or health services with reference to self-help groups are never justified.
>
> (Trogan 1989: 231)

If confirmed by subsequent research, self-help groups would be valued for their emancipating effects, improvement in quality of life, and their ability to bring about change in the type and range of services that are provided. At present it does not look as though they actually reduce demands on mainstream services.

THE ROLE OF OTHER INDIVIDUALS IN SUPPORTING SELF-CARE

In contrast to professional care, support for self-care from others is likely to be predicated on mutual indebtedness stemming from social ties. This is captured in anthropological notions of 'gift exchange' and 'altruism'. These suggest that moral obligation and reciprocity are the basis of informal care to others. This creates patterns of reciprocity with 'gift giving' serving as the mechanism by which people commence and sustain social relationships (Komter 1996). The reciprocity upon which patterns of lay care appear to be based is not equitably distributed. Those whose needs are greatest tend to receive the least because reciprocity is dependent on access to personal, social and emotional resources to reciprocate. There is evidence in the area of informal health care that those who most need to be reciprocal, and to meet others' needs, have the fewest resources to do so (Arber and Ginn 1992).

Elements of the nature of reciprocity and the involvement of others were evident in the accounts provided in our 'Pathways to Care' study. Where there was more than one person in the household, support and self-care was sometimes reinforcing. This is evident in this example where an elderly couple suffer from the same condition. Mutual support is evident from the wife's account of her own and her husband's arthritis:

> *Respondent:* *I mean he's the same, he's got it in his neck. It's funny, I've got it all down my left side and he's got his down his right side so we say, we're laughing at home and we'll say we could do with having half and half cutting one another in two and heaving the good half and the bad half . . .*
>
> *Interviewer:* *Do you find it helps living with somebody who's got similar things?*
>
> *Respondent:* *Well yes, because you can sympathize with one another . . .*

The capacity and willingness of other people to substitute work tasks are also important in the success or otherwise of individuals' attempts at self-care. This is illustrated with reference to two people who had been diagnosed with musculoskeletal complaints and whose efforts at self-care depended on their ability to manoeuvre the routines of work. The first, a retired man, described the way in which he managed and controlled his arthritis in a way which prevented him from going to the doctors:

> *Well I don't do any hard work, any lifting or nothing like that, because if I do that then it will set if off because the discs have wasted away.*

Different contingencies came into play for this woman, who had had major surgery on her back. Her knowledge about what should be done (i.e. avoiding lifting) was sabotaged by the events and context of her paid work as a care assistant. This placed her in a position where she could not avoid lifting and subsequently resulted in a consultation with her GP:

> *The RGN I was on with and the other girl are both pregnant, and I work in a nursing home so it was a case of, 'Well we can't do anything, we can't pick up a piece of paper off the floor, we're pregnant!' Oh great. Well I had one lady that fell three times in one night, so it was a case of getting her up off the floor and you couldn't get the hoist in the bedroom so I had to do it myself.*

This contrasted with the experience of another respondent who was a care assistant who reported being able to rely on the positive relationship that had developed between herself and her work colleagues:

> *I work nights and we're a good staff together. If I was having a bad night they would help me out, have a night off if I was really bad.*

In our pathways study, the support, indebtedness, and the way in which it was repaid differed according to a number of factors, including type and stability of social networks. Those people who worked tended to identify key support networks across work and domestic settings. The type of support differed. Middle-class respondents were more likely than working-class respondents to have access to formal or quasi-formal health knowledge gained through the expertise or experience of those in their social networks. They were also more likely to identify professionals as forming part of their networks. The status of this knowledge (coming from professional health workers) at times acted as ammunition when there were doubts about the medical explanation and information provided by the GP.

Instrumental support, based on contact rather than knowledge, was more evident where access to material and social resources was limited. In this regard, some accounts fitted more with a traditional view of kinship ties and relationships of obligation and exchange. In the example below, this related to neighbours/friends who were seen on a daily basis. Locality and tight social ties were described in this account when discussing information and informal support around health matters:

> *Well I call on my mum and dad because they are parents, and P and T next door . . . then a father, daughter and a son M down the road. There is about three or four of us who normally can talk through the day.*

The reciprocity or exchange of support generated by close proximity is illustrated by this description in which concerns about a shortage of money and access to resources predominate:

> *When he had his last by-pass done, his wife slipped when it was bad you know at winter and he said, 'I've got to go up to the top shop.' I said, 'Oh well, don't walk up,' I said, 'I've got the car now, I'll run you' . . . and he said, 'I'll give you some money for petrol.' I said, 'Don't be daft.' Because county was on in a couple of weeks wasn't they – on Sky . . . and we can't tune into the channel it was on, and he said, 'Come over and watch the match with me.'*

SELF- AND PROFESSIONAL CARE: THE BASIS OF A SHARED AGENDA?

Professional care has been described as affectively instrumental, specialized, neutral and impersonal. Lay care, in contrast, is depicted as being characterized by emotional support and care based on personal experience (Dean 1986). However, this distinction hides a convergence of the philosophy of care in the lay and professional worlds. Affective and holistic care have increasingly been claimed as part of nursing and primary care work (Williams *et al.* 1997). Similarly, as we discussed in Chapter 4, lay knowledge is imbued with, and incorporates, aspects of medical knowledge and care. Some individuals, particularly those with long-term illnesses or psychosocial problems may look to professionals for primarily interpersonal contact. This may be a more valued aspect of health care than the possession of technical skills (Bendtsen *et al.* 1995). Thus, while some researchers consider there to be a clear-cut distinction between self-care and professional care, others view self-care and professional care as a continuum.

A focus on aspects of disease management involving lay care activities as well as professional care and self-care activities is influenced to a large extent by professional health services contact. Additionally, contemporary self-care practices are swayed to a large extent by a diffuse set of cultural influences and resources. These lie beyond the confines of health professionals and services. As we shall see in Chapter 8, both formal and informal information sources are important in disseminating knowledge about health and illness. However, the ways in which professional and lay worlds meet, in productive dialogue or unproductive opposition, around the benefits and limitations of self-care, are likely to influence the type and nature of the latter.

The views of professionals about self-care appear to be ambivalent. There are conditions, such as asthma and diabetes, in which self-management is encouraged as a central part of treatment. In these realms, professionals have actively tried to shape and control self-management strategies adopted by individuals and their families (Mesters *et al.* 1991). Additionally, self-help groups have been more readily accepted as complementing professional care. A recent study found mainly positive professional attitudes about the effectiveness, merits and functions of lay help groups. Predominant characteristics of successful partnerships were identified by professionals as equality, flexibility, decreased professional control, mutual understanding and shared goals. The major obstacles to partnerships were seen to be poor communication, negative attitudes, role ambiguity, the limits of the health care system and ideological conflicts (Stewart *et al.* 1995). However, the conclusion of a review of professionals' views of self-care carried out in the 1980s indicated 'considerable variation among physicians in their attitudes and perceptions: these have been found to be a function of their professional training and practice experience as well as of a variety of personal attributes'. Generally, self-care is seen by GPs as having the potential to reduce formal health care consultations and the costs of health care. However, self-care practices in which patients express independence and question the physician's authority may be perceived with hostility (Shuval *et al.* 1989). Compared with lay people's own assessments, professionals have been found to underestimate lay capabilities in relation to psychosocial and self-care aspects of their care (Vanagthoven and Plomp 1989) and there is a tendency for health professionals to see themselves as superior in knowledge about self-care (Vincent 1992). Research on professional views of self-help groups suggests that community health workers may be sympathetic to the idea of alternative and self-help but there was also anxiety about threats to their professional authority. The same research showed a lack of awareness of the range of self-help groups and self-care strategies that were available to people (Unell 1986).

The interaction of lay and professional worlds in decisions and enquiries about appropriate health care was evident from the qualitative interviews in the 'Pathways to Care' study. At times, the impact of medical authority on people's willingness to consider alternatives suggests that the medical profession is highly influential in being able to direct self-care in relation to certain population groups. The impact of medical authority and willingness of individuals to accept it is illustrated by this elderly man's account given in response to being asked whether he used any alternative therapies or home remedies:

> *No not really. I've read about them; I mean you read these articles in the Reader's Digest and things like that about these various sorts of things, but no, I believe that if you are going to the doctor's you should be doing what he tells you and not doing something that you are not telling him about. That's the important thing . . . it might be leading you in a different direction to what you really should be going in and if you are not telling him then he might think it's the medicine he's giving you.*

However, this man did take garlic tablets for his heart because they were given to him by the occupational health department. He says he sticks to what the doctor tells him because otherwise there is no point in going to the doctor and the patient has a *duty* to take the prescribed medications. In another instance, a friend's advice about visiting a herbalist was not acted upon 'because of the doctors', and a middle-aged woman living on her own said she did not consider self-care because she only takes medicines if given advice by a doctor or chemist.

One woman started taking evening primrose oil for her bones, but stopped because she felt she no longer needed to take it after her doctor diagnosed osteoporosis and prescribed her medication (Posamax): 'I feel what the doctor has prescribed for me should work for me.' Fear of counteracting allopathic medicine prescribed from formal sources was also a reason for not trying home remedies but relying on services. One elderly man with bronchitis said that he did not try alternative therapies because he was happy with the drugs he took and was concerned that if he mixed things they might knock him back.

The influence of medical authority was also evident in the accounts people gave of their everyday care regimes they undertook for themselves. This example of a husband and wife who both had arthritis is an example of how self-care practices are often a mixture of home-grown self-care measures and 'doctor's orders':

Interviewer:	*So how do you try to cope with your arthritis then apart from your medication? What do you do?*
Respondent (woman):	*You've got to cope to forget the pains.*
Interviewer:	*Do you do anything to relieve it yourself?*
Respondent (man):	*Have a walk out.*
Respondent (woman):	*I do sewing, I do a lot of sewing. Do you know these? I've made all these [pointing to embroidery]. If I get the pains in my knees and I'm sat down I've got to get up and walk about.*
Respondent (man):	*And she has warm baths as well.*
Respondent (woman):	*It's what my doctor told me to do otherwise they will seize up.*
Interviewer:	*And is there anything else you do to relieve it, to ease the pain?*
Respondent (man):	*I put cream on it or a gel and take my pain killers.*
Interviewer:	*And is that all from your doctor that?*
Respondent (man):	*Yeah.*

However, medical authority, either as a promoter or retarder of self-care practices, was less evident in younger age groups, where knowledge about alternative practices raised questions for people about the legitimacy of the advice and treatment provided in primary care. A woman who consulted her GP for a health problem did so against a household context in which family members had gained information about alternatives and had used them for a variety of ailments, and where the possibility of the utility and use of alternatives arose as a legitimate possibility that her GP should consider. Her husband had used osteopathy for a back problem when he had lost the feeling in his legs. Her mother-in-law regularly used homeopathy and aromatherapy and she had tried homeopathic medicine from the pharmacist for a mouth problem. She took yeast and Olbas oil regularly for sinus trouble:

> *GPs don't really like all this alternative medicine, but there are some adapting to it now, you know what I mean, and trying to play alongside it, go hand in hand together ... but he said, 'You've got mild arthritis in your neck that could have been causing all the headaches and that and it's from your neck going up into your head', and I said, 'Oh well, what can I do now to help that?' He said, 'What?' I said, 'This arthritis.' I thought arthritis from what I could see ... old ladies, and I thought, What can I do? 'Well there's nothing you can do', and I said, 'Nothing like cod liver oil or anything?', and he went, 'No', and that was it.*

In discussing the issue of providing information to patients she returned to the issue:

> *Maybe the doctor should say to you like, 'Well there's nothing, no there's nothing within us that can do it but, err, you should, there might be something homeopathic, you can get your infor-mation here or there.*

Being aware of the range and diversity of attitudes to self-care is relevant for encouraging mutual understanding between pro-fessionals and patients. Managed self-care programmes of common ailments presented to primary care have occasionally been evalu-ated by clinical trials. The results are equivocal. A study by Kiely and McPherson (1986) compared people who had received a self-administered stress package, given during a consultation with a GP, with those receiving GP consultation alone. The study showed a modest reduction in symptoms and consulting rates in those who had used the packages. With regard to chronic headaches, a self-care programme[4] was found to be more successful than GP consul-tation alone, and treatment gains increased over time (Winkler *et al.* 1989). However, two factors from this latter study highlight the limitations for managing demand through self-care in real-life situ-ations. First, 'the data were not consistent with a strong claim that a self-care programme, such as the one used in the study, substan-tially reduced health costs, at least in the case of chronic headaches in general practice'. Second, and more important, is the high non-acceptance among those referred to the self-care programme. The researchers concluded that 'the high non-acceptance among those referred suggests that the widespread promulgation of self-care

approaches in primary care may meet with some patient resistance'
(Winkler *et al.* 1989: 219). Thus the implementation of evidence-
based packages of care may not reach those who are likely to gain
most from them.

SUMMARY

Over the last two decades self-care has emerged as a solution to
many of the problems of highly medicalized and resource-limited
health care systems. It has held out the hope of reducing iatrogenic
illness, lessening dependence on medical authority and slowing
down rising health care costs. While the impact of the self-care
movement should not be underestimated, in relation to bringing
about positive cultural change in the way in which patients are
viewed, there is as yet little unequivocal evidence to support the
notion that self-care reduces the overall demand for formal health
care services. However, the potential for responding to need more
effectively is likely to be influenced by the self-care strategies which
people undertake for themselves. Central to devising sensitive services is a professional recognition of the self-care people already
undertake for themselves and ensuring that service response com-
pliments rather than contradicts these efforts. Professionals might
gain from understanding the complexities of the content and
process of self-care so that formal services can be fitted to what
patients are already doing for themselves.

The relevant literature reviewed and our own research suggest
that self-care encompasses a wide range of everyday habitual action
on the part of individuals. The cost, effectiveness and acceptability
of self-care resources are important determinants of their utilization. The practices, beliefs and views of lay people are varied and
these variations occur both within and between social groups. Thus,
consciousness raising about self-care practices from official health
sources may be perceived and responded to in a variety of ways. A
negative reaction about the principle of self-care may be found
among some population groups, particularly those with a high
regard for medical knowledge. Those who do not undertake self-
care activities, or resist it being suggested, need to be considered as
a different population from those who embrace self-care. The
demand for, and the appropriate content of, primary health care
interventions are likely to be different for the two groups. The promotion of self-care practices will need to acknowledge the scope

and meanings which individuals attach to such activities if promotional campaigns and materials are to be acceptable and appropriate to those who will use them. Primary health care professional attitudes towards, and knowledge of, healing practices which fall outside traditional allopathic medicine will also affect how demand is met. This may require a re-evaluation of the way in which patients' autonomy and knowledge about health care matters is construed at an individual level. It also begs questions about the skill-base of contemporary primary care professionals in understanding the range and extent of lay knowledge and lay action about health. Self-care is not only about the interface between individual patient activity and professional care but is also about the social, psychological and material resources which shape these activities. Access to these will influence the extent and the way in which people can and do take more or less responsibility for their health.

NOTES

1 At times the focus on symptoms seems to be at the expense of ascertaining the reasons for non-action, and for most of the clinical iceberg-type studies the reasons for non-action are not the subject of exploration with subjects.
2 An American study by Thompson *et al.* (1993) suggests that in relation to some illnesses, such as cancer, it is more important for patients to believe that they can control daily emotional reactions and physical symptoms than the course of the disease.
3 In the study by Wadsworth *et al.* (1971) for example, the use of home remedies was incorporated in the 'other' category, which accounted for less than 1 per cent of all treatment and consultation activity. Similarly, 20 years later, secondary analysis of US illness behaviour data, which was not specifically collected for the analysis of self-care, found that only 5 per cent of illness responses were self-treatments (Giachello *et al.* 1982). In this latter study the options for home treatments from which respondents could choose only included the use of diets and appliances, so excluding a number of other forms of self-care.
4 The self-care programme emphasized active patient participation using stress management, and focused on teaching patients skills for use in the control of headache episodes through relaxation training (and cognitive restructuring) and the management of lifestyle factors that precipitated or aggravated headaches.

PART III

MEDIATING DEMAND IN PRIMARY CARE

7

COMMUNITY PHARMACY AS A PRIMARY CARE AND A SELF-CARE RESOURCE

Many persons ... object to calling in a medical man on every trivial occasion. They resort to their own nostrums and family receipts, and in the application of these remedies the Chemist is sometimes consulted, not as a medical man, but as a person who, from his constant manipulation of medicines, is supposed to know something about their effects.
(Jacob Bell, quoted in *Royal Pharmaceutical Society of Great Britain 1841–1991. A Political and Social History*)

The early nineteenth-century chemist and druggist were the providers of primary health care for the whole population.
(Holloway, *Royal Pharmaceutical Society of Great Britain 1841–1991. A Political and Social History*)

INTRODUCTION

This chapter focuses on the underacknowledged part that community pharmacy staff play in primary care in mediating demand and reinforcing patients' own self-care behaviour. Community pharmacies operate across the interface between informal care networks and formal primary care provision, but it is only recently that researchers have begun to explore and clarify the particular manner in which individuals use pharmacy staff as one of a number of resources in response to an illness episode. As we saw in Chapter 6, self-medication is one of the most common responses to minor illness, but the role pharmacies and pharmacy staff play in providing this medication is relatively underexplored. Currently with free medical consultations and an 85 per cent level of exemption from prescription charges, relief from minor ailments is being sought from GPs. The government is keen to shift this demand by making community pharmacies 'the first port of call' for minor ailments, and reduce the consultation workload and prescribing costs on GPs for trivial complaints.

The first part of the chapter draws together findings from relevant literature to describe patterns and rates of pharmacy use. The second part examines the different ways in which individuals utilize pharmacies as a primary health care and self-care resource by focusing on an analysis of data from a qualitative pharmacy study (see Appendix for further details) which set out to explore the manner, the nature and the process of advice giving and advice seeking from pharmacies. Data from the 'Pathways to Care' study is also drawn upon. In the wider context of the book the manner in which the issue of demand for pharmacy services has been formulated is examined and questions about how organizational and other factors may influence demand for, and use of, pharmacy services are considered.

PATTERNS OF PHARMACY CONSULTATIONS

Generally, women make more use of pharmacies than men, with females accounting for anywhere between 60 per cent and 80 per cent of customers (Hardisty 1982; Mottram *et al.* 1989; Hayes and Livingstone 1990; Smith 1992). In particular, women with small children are more likely to consult pharmacy staff, and individuals with chronic illnesses (e.g. diabetics, coeliacs) have also been identified as high pharmacy users (Jepson *et al.* 1991). Men use pharmacies infrequently, especially those in full-time employment, and those aged 16–24 (Tully and Temple 1997). In general 'elderly' people are frequent or high users (Hayes and Livingstone 1990; Jepson *et al.* 1991), but their high use is restricted mostly to the prescription service (RPSGB 1996), while the very elderly (over 75-year-olds) have been identified as low users (Tully and Temple 1997). Low levels of pharmacy use among the very elderly is probably related to mobility, but low use of pharmacies by the elderly for general health advice (Fisher *et al.* 1991; Whittaker *et al.* 1995) is thought to be related to their greater need for medical attention, such that pharmacies are a less feasible alternative for them (Ritchie *et al.* 1981). Their belief in the general practitioner as the only health professional with the legitimate expertise to diagnose and treat them is thought likely to explain part of their reluctance to use pharmacies as a primary health care resource (Livingstone 1995).

Only two studies examine how ethnic minority communities use community pharmacy services (Jesson *et al.* 1994). One small West Midlands study found that Asian respondents were unlikely to visit a pharmacist for advice, while few visited a pharmacy even for OTC medicines. Similarly, the larger consumer expectations survey (Jesson *et al.* 1994) found that while ethnic minority customers were aware of the pharmacist's advisory role, they did not use it very much. Their low consultation rates again appeared to be related to their perception that the community pharmacist was not viewed as an appropriate person to ask for advice on symptoms of ill health or general health issues. Instead, the doctor was viewed as the most appropriate person to consult.

Studies on the symptoms and conditions presented by patients in pharmacies show that the range is very broad. Most are minor self-limiting ailments, rather than more general or more serious 'health problems'. Respiratory ailments, gastro-intestinal complaints and skin conditions are among the most common complaints presented (Smith 1992; McElnay and Dickson 1994).

THE EXTENT OF PHARMACY USE

Frequency of pharmacy use is high, and in general, people visit their pharmacy more frequently than their GP. Over 65 per cent of the public visit a pharmacy at least once a month (McElnay *et al.* 1993), while between 80 per cent and 94 per cent of the population visit their pharmacy at least once a year (Jepson *et al.* 1991; RPSGB 1996; Tully and Temple 1997). The proportion visiting their GP this often is around 78 per cent (OPCS 1995).

Despite professional and government policy supporting the use of pharmacies as the 'first port of call' for the treatment of minor illness (DoH 1996), existing research literature suggests that the extent of the public's use of pharmacies as a first response to minor ailments is not large. The core service most frequently used in pharmacies is the prescription medication supply service. Two recent studies (RPSGB 1996; Tully and Temple 1997), for example, showed that over 80 per cent of people who had visited their pharmacy in the last 12 months had done so in order to get a prescription. By contrast, visiting a pharmacy for advice on a minor ailment or more general health care advice is still quite rare, with most individuals, when professional care or advice is sought, seeking care from a GP in preference to any other health professional. Pharmacy studies present evidence that people are more likely to seek advice from their pharmacist rather than their GP for only three named common ailments (ticklish cough; minor eye irritation; hay fever) (Mottram *et al.* 1989; John *et al.* 1995). In the case of advice for more indeterminate conditions it has been estimated that between 2 per cent and 15 per cent choose pharmacies instead of a GP (Ritchie *et al.* 1981; Cunningham-Burley and Maclean 1987; Morrow *et al.* 1993; Kayne and Reeves 1994; Cantrill *et al.* 1996; RPSGB 1996).

THE NATURE OF PHARMACY USE

Interviews with individuals in the 'Pathways to Care' study who recorded having used the pharmacy reveal some interesting insights into how people decide to seek care from the pharmacy rather than their GP. These interviews suggest that pharmacies are used mostly as another self-care resource. While some individuals see pharmacy use as a suitable alternative to the GP, it is only for the treatment of minor ailments, and in most cases they have already decided before entering the pharmacy which medicine to purchase to treat the illness they themselves have already diagnosed. Pharmacy staff are being used for reassurance and as an avenue of referral to the GP, rather than as health professionals with a role in primary care recognized by the public.

Pharmacists as an alternative to the GP

When individuals decide to use the pharmacy instead of the GP, the decision appears to be linked to lay notions of what constitutes inappropriate use of general practitioners. Studies by social scientists on the nature of use of general practice have noted that people do make clear distinctions about which service it is appropriate to use for certain complaints, such that for conditions perceived as serious, a visit to the GP is their first choice (Cartwright and Smith 1988; Wyke *et al.* 1990). For minor ailments, on the other hand, pharmacists are viewed as an alternative to the GP. For some they are seen as a more suitable choice because of their own special expertise, but for most it was because they considered the GP's time too valuable to waste (Hassell *et al.* 1997a). The refrain: 'I didn't want to bother the doctor' was articulated by many of the pharmacy users interviewed in the NPCRDC studies:

I don't trouble the doctor unless I particularly have to, and, if, you know, generally, if it was just minor things I just go to the chemist and ask for them.

If it was something minor, you know, sort of an everyday ailment, I would be more likely to ask the pharmacist.

I might defer going to the doctors if the situation wasn't serious.

Familiarity with and persistence of the complaint are also key features in choosing between the two services. If individuals have suffered before with the ailment and consider it 'common', 'trivial' or 'minor' they are more likely to use the pharmacy, while a 'major' or 'serious' matter merits a visit to the GP. Most people, however, relate their use of pharmacies to matters of convenience:

. . . it's more convenient to nip in the chemist and say, 'Have you got something for this cough?'

Particularly for those who work a visit to the pharmacy is much more convenient, mostly because obtaining GP appointments and waiting in busy surgeries can be burdensome:

Well, it's usually if somebody's ill and with working full-time you see, you can't always get an appointment to see the doctor when it's convenient, until the weekend. So if somebody's ill I'll go in and have a word with him and say, 'What do you recommend?', but if it's serious, he will say, 'Well you really need to get to the doctor . . .'

For many, however, use of pharmacies as an alternative is tied up with the view that GPs' time is more important, perhaps more highly valued, than that of pharmacists. The following woman felt that by taking up an appointment for a trivial complaint she would be 'bothering' her GP, and would be preventing people with more urgent needs from seeing the doctor:

I just feel that you go to the doctor's when you . . . are ill, you know what I mean. I mean some people are always going to the doctor's aren't they, for tiny bits of things, and I just thought it wasn't worth troubling the doctor over, because taking up an appointment for somebody that probably was quite ill and would need the appointment. That's how I look at it.

> *It's usually the best place to go before you go bothering the doctor, you know.*

We highlighted in Chapter 4 the relationship between past service use and how experiences of disillusionment with professional care can be responsible for failure to seek medical help in the future. It is also the case that a previous poor experience with one service will encourage people to seek care from alternative services. Others have noted previously that people sometimes prefer the pharmacist because they are dissatisfied with the treatment or medication prescribed by their doctor, or because the pharmacy staff are viewed as more helpful and the doctor unsympathetic (Ritchie *et al.* 1981; Cunningham-Burley and Maclean 1987; Hassell *et al.* 1997). There was also evidence from several people in the 'Pathways to Care' study that pharmacists are sometimes preferred because of a dissatisfaction with their GP:

> *With regards to the children's colds, I think you're probably dealt with more sympathetically by the pharmacist because the doctors, they're seeing so many children that go through, you know, with sore throats, etc., that I think, particularly in the village, the doctor's very much, well, do you want antibiotics, Calpol . . . yet taking the advice of the pharmacist, buying the product they suggested, by the next day, his symptoms, you know, he was a different child again. Whereas the doctor's advice had just been Calpol, which really was not helping him at all.*

The following woman preferred the pharmacist, because he provided her with more detailed information. In part, this appeared to be associated with her perception that the GP does not have sufficient time to talk, and by implication the pharmacist does:

> *You get more information off the pharmacist because naturally he knows a lot about the drugs that you are taking. The doctor will give you the pills but unless you ask him, and of course he hasn't got much time to explain, you want to know what that tablet is going to do to you, what it is actually for. Sometimes they will just give you, now I was given some, when I went with my sciatica first of all, he gave me some tablets and that was it, I'd been taking some tablets that were more or less the same, and he said, 'No these are stronger', so I went to the pharmacist and I said, 'What actually do these tablets do?' He said, 'Well it's for*

the inflammation, to take the inflammation down', which the doctor hadn't explained to me, so of course naturally I was all right, I knew what they were going to do, what they were actually for, they were like Nurofen but they were a bit stronger, because when it said Nurofen I looked on the thing and said, 'Oh I've been taking Nurofen, doctor', and he said, 'Oh these are like them but a bit stronger', but he didn't actually say what they were going to do, he said, 'It will stop the pain', but he didn't actually say what they do to stop the pain.

Pharmacists as a self-care resource

In the pharmacy observation study, requests for advice or treatment based on the description of symptoms to pharmacy staff by pharmacy customers were not as common as were demands for named products. The latter were a significant feature of pharmacy/client interactions in this study, suggesting that a large proportion of the public know what they want to purchase for their minor ailment well before they reach the pharmacy. They have already diagnosed their illness, and are effectively dealing with the purchase of the remedy in much the same way as the purchase of any other commodity.

Other customers presented with symptoms instead of demanding named products. These customers often seek a product recommendation, but occasionally they seek reassurance from the pharmacy assistants or the pharmacist. This may be reassurance about the action they intend to take; it may be that their medication is correct, that they are taking it correctly, that it will do them no harm, and, strangely, that it might actually do them some good. Such customers will pepper the discourse with 'Is it any good?', suggesting that these customers are concerned with the *effectiveness* of the medication:

Customer:	*What have you got for a sore throat?*
Pharmacy Assistant:	*Is it for you?*
Customer:	*Yes [sniffing loudly].*
Pharmacy Assistant:	*These are Bradasol sugar free, or do you want a stronger one? These are strong [reading pack]: one every two to three hours. No more than eight in a day and do not drink or eat for one hour.*
Customer:	*That's no good then.*

> Pharmacy Assistant: Or there's these – Decquadin.
> Customer: Are these good?
>   [Pharmacist joins conversation]
> Pharmacist: Yes.
> Customer: Right.

Use of pharmacies by the public also differs from the use of GP services in relation to the proportion of 'proxy' patients. In general practice it is unusual for doctors to see patients who visit on behalf of other individuals, but in pharmacy the extent of 'proxy' use is relatively high, with studies reporting around 27 per cent and 30 per cent of pharmacy visitors purchasing medicines or asking advice for other people. Another study looking at how pharmacists deal with patients presenting with cough symptoms reported that 43 per cent were consulting for someone else, usually a child. Although individuals in the two pharmacy studies here did not make any explicit observations themselves about the benefit of using pharmacies to get advice or reassurance for other people, direct observations of pharmacy staff and client interactions demonstrated and reinforced findings from other studies, that proxy use of pharmacy services is high. While the opportunity to seek advice on behalf of a third party is a major benefit of using pharmacies, and may indirectly shape demand for the services, the following exchange between a proxy customer and pharmacy staff nevertheless demonstrates the difficulties staff sometimes experience when trying to determine the appropriateness of a purchase for someone not present in the pharmacy:

> Male (aged 20 yrs): I want some Contac 400.
> Pharmacy Assistant: Are they for you?
> Male: No. Girlfriend.
> Assistant: Is she on any other medication?
> Male: I don't know. I don't think so.
> Assistant: Just check with her will you [putting product in bag].

It is perhaps paradoxical that while pharmacies provide easy access to advice on minor ailments to the public, especially carers, advice by proxy is one of the most difficult parts of the pharmacist's job, often because the proxy simply does not have access to the sort of information the pharmacist believes he or she needs to make a suitable treatment suggestion as indicated by this quote from one community pharmacist:

The difficulty is when you're not speaking to the person you want to treat, and that does happen a significant amount. When somebody is coming in for somebody else, whether it's for their elderly mother or the neighbour or whoever. And that's more difficult, but all you can do is really ask as many questions and get as good a feel for the situation as you can.

Pharmacists as agents of referral

In a study conducted in the early eighties, Cunningham-Burley and Maclean (1987) identified that pharmacists are discriminating in the way that they identify medical problems and what should be done with them. The National Primary Care Research and Development Centre (NPCRDC) pharmacy observation study (Hassell *et al.* 1996) found similar evidence, although the extent to which the task of differentiating between problems occurred was not extensive (only 6 per cent of customers purchasing OTC products were referred to their GP or other service). Nevertheless, some pharmacy clients view pharmacists as a 'stepping stone' to general practice (Hassell *et al.* 1997). The referral function is reassuring, and acts as a safety net between their own care action (as advised by the pharmacist or not as the case may be) and the GP. It is often seen as a valued and important aspect of the pharmactist's role, with customers revealing an *expectation* that pharmacy staff are there to refer them on when necessary:

. . . if she can't tell me she says, 'You better ask your doctor'. So obviously she's not fobbing you off with, you know, just her own ideas. She'll tell you straight if she doesn't really know, or if she feels it's better that you should see your doctor . . .

. . . sometimes if a GP is busy, you don't like trivial questions. You are asking him these questions which sound trivial, and then you know he could be seeing another patient. So, you know, the pharmacist, when you get the prescription are quite helpful, and if need be they recommend you back to the doctor – that's what the lady did last time.

There appears to be wide variation in the proportion of pharmacy customers referred on to their GP. Some observation studies have identified as few as 5 per cent and 6 per cent of pharmacy clients being referred on to their doctor (Mukerjee and Blane 1990; Hassell *et al.* 1997), while other studies have reported rates of 40 per cent and 45 per cent (Evans *et al.* 1996; Krska and Kennedy 1996). Several authors suggest that referral patterns are mostly determined by characteristics of symptoms presented, so that the more serious a complaint seems, the more likely the patient will be referred (Smith 1993; Hassell *et al.* 1996). The availability of suitable OTC products to treat the conditions presented, and the pharmacists' own skills, are also likely to affect the rate of referrals to GPs and other health care professionals (Hassell *et al.* 1997).

The pharmacy observational study suggested that several criteria are important in the decisions that pharmacists make in relation to referring on to general practice or other services. The *seriousness* of the ailment appeared important. Pharmacists discriminated according to the potential severity of the problem encountered, such that, for example, the majority of referrals concerned problems with infected eyes, persistent coughs, gastro-intestinal or skin complaints. In instances when a suitable OTC product was not available to treat the condition, the pharmacist would refer to the GP, but pharmacists' own risk management also involved a 'play safe' attitude which meant that in situations of doubt or uncertainty they would refer a client to his or her GP:

> *It depends on the symptoms you're treating . . . if it's a straightforward self-limiting ailment then that's actually quite straightforward to deal with. If it's a . . . if there are other things that provide question marks in your own mind, then you refer.*

PATIENT FACTORS WHICH INFLUENCE DEMAND FOR PHARMACY CARE

The concept of 'approachability' has been applied to pharmacists, such that they are considered to be less socially removed from their customers than doctors, and less formal. This is thought to make them less threatening and more amenable to the majority of the public (Cunningham-Burley and Maclean 1987; Bissell *et al.* 1996). The finding, from a London-based study, that over two-thirds of customers used pharmacies because of the lack of obligation to take advice reinforces this idea (Smith 1990a). This quality may be particularly important for certain groups of clients, for example, drug addicts, who would otherwise be lost to medical services (Mulleady and Green 1985). In one study about pharmacy needle exchange, 49 per cent of clients were drug users not in contact with other health-related services, such that pharmacy-based schemes were said by clients to provide a convenient alternative to agency needle exchange schemes without compromising user confidentiality. That pharmacies might be used when medical care is not available or accessible is an important consideration in relation to access to primary care services and issues around equality of provision, but has so far been the subject of only a few studies (Mukerjee and Blane 1990).

While some consumers of health care view the pharmacist as a suitable alternative to the GP, there is evidence to suggest that perceptions by consumers of the professional boundaries and responsibilities of different professional groups may account for why others do not see the pharmacist fulfilling a formal primary care role. The following woman clearly believed that it is not the pharmacist's area of expertise and responsibility to diagnose illness:

> . . . *and I don't begrudge paying like a couple of quid for a bottle of medicine for them, but no, I tend to ask the doctor's advice because I think I could be purchasing the wrong thing; or the chemist doesn't look down his throat, check his ears, check his stomach, and things like that. Plus the doctor knows our medical history.*

Thus, while customers are generally very satisfied with pharmacy services (for example, see Morrow *et al.* 1993; Kayne and Reeves 1994; Krska *et al.* 1994), the fairly widely held belief that pharmacists cannot or do not diagnose may go some way to explaining the low level of use of the pharmacy as the first port of call for treatment or advice about minor ailments.

Consumer perception about differences in professional responsibilities is also shaped by differences in the way GPs and pharmacies operate regarding access to medical records and patients' medical history. In the 'Pathways to Care' study several people on regular prescription medicines for serious illnesses believed that the doctor was the best person to go to because of his/her familiarity with their medical history:

> *Well the doctor has got all your records there and they know what you can and can't have. I mean the pharmacist could give me something that might react to my other stuff.*

The pharmacy customer interviews also demonstrated the degree to which individuals weigh up the cost (financial and physical) and benefit of seeking pharmacy or medical care. In the context of prescription prices and deregulation of prescription-only medicines, there is evidence to suggest that cost may be a factor in determining whether individuals use the pharmacy instead of general practice (Cunningham-Burley and Maclean 1987; Cartwright and Smith 1988; McElnay and Dickson 1994; Hassell *et al.* 1996; Payne *et al.* 1996; Schafheutle *et al.* 1996). When OTC products are cheaper than a prescription some consumers will visit the pharmacy instead of the doctor (Cartwright and Smith 1988; McElnay and Dickson 1994; Hassell *et al.* 1996; Schafheutle *et al.* 1996). Others who receive free prescriptions may have little choice but to visit the GP. The cost of medicines was the driving force behind the pattern of this young woman's use of primary health care services. She preferred the pharmacist's advice about the medication she should use, but a GP consultation was necessary as well because of the cost of the product she needed for her children:

> *I mean if they [her children] have got a cold or something like that, I would probably ask them [pharmacy staff] what is the best one for a cold, but most probably go to the doctor's [to get a prescription] because you don't have to, you don't need to pay from the doctor's.*

Similarly, another young mother of two toddlers said:

> *I suppose that's why I take them to the doctor's more, so I can get the prescription rather than getting the cough medicine and the Calpol and stuff over the counter.*

This attitude was not uncommon. Another woman said she never visits the chemist, but always goes to the doctor when she is ill because:

> *. . . you have to pay at the chemist . . . Well, the colds stuff, it can be expensive can't it, so you know, why pay when you can get it free? [laughs]*

Prescription exemption status, however, does not mean all clients will always use their GP. The cost of OTC and prescription medicines and convenience issues are inter-related and impact differently on different groups of people. Some people also perceive the cost issue in relation to judgements about appropriateness again. This pensioner, living in an affluent, rural area, despite being exempt from prescription charges, was happy to pay for some drugs:

> *I don't try to get painkillers or anything like that really, to save me money. I mean the necessary drugs I'm very happy to have on prescription, because for all I know the beta blockers may be quite expensive, I don't know. But I mean to go and ask the doctor if I can have some paracetamol I think is a bit much, so I pay for those myself.*

It is possible that the low level of demand for the advisory aspect of the pharmacy service is related to a lack of need for the service. Prior experience of the symptoms (Smith 1990b), previous use of the product (McElnay and Dickson 1994), or the fact that advice had already been given (by other health care professionals or family and friends) (Elliot-Binns 1973; Cartwright and Smith 1988; Oakley 1994; Livingstone 1995) are all likely to reduce individuals' need to seek pharmacy advice on how to take medication or on the treatment of minor ailments.

The nature of pharmacy use is also likely to be shaped by lay attitudes to medicines. Blaxter and Britten (1996) recently noted that a better knowledge of lay attitudes to medicines would be of considerable value to pharmacy practice, but it is an area which has received little attention. Evidence from the latest NPCRDC pharmacy study indicates that while the purchase of OTCs from pharmacies and their use is high, some individuals perceive OTC and prescription medicines differently. Pharmacy thus has its limits. While OTCs can help control pain, consumers' concerns about immunity as a result of long-term use and the strength of OTC against prescription remedies affect the extent to which pharmacies are likely to be used. In particular, beliefs about the effectiveness of OTC medicines are likely to determine whether individuals self-medicate or seek a GP consultation (Hassell *et al.* forthcoming). This 59-year-old woman, when asked about medicines, said:

> *. . . you can be on a certain tablet for so long and they don't have any effect on you. You need a change.*

Later on in the interview she mentioned an OTC cough product she had tried and when asked what she thought about it she replied:

> *Sometimes they, they don't have any effect . . . you are better off going and getting one from, what she [the doctor] prescribes . . . I mean you can have a Veno's one and they don't work all the time.*

A young woman with a history of bad headaches had tried OTC products for some time. The symptoms did not improve and eventually she went to her GP for a 'stronger' medicine: *'it's one of the strongest ones he can give me'*. However, she still has headaches and she now puts this down to being immune to their effect because of the length of time she has taken them:

> *I took the tablets but I got immune to them. With having a constant headache I'd take four or five and it wasn't going away.*

A person's previous medical history will also impact on the manner in which they make use of community pharmacy services. This very active 74-year-old woman, while very satisfied with her local pharmacy and the staff, was adamant she would never ask the pharmacist for advice:

> *No, I would not. I would go to the doctor. Well, I can't afford to take chances because of my medical history. I just go straight away.*

The same was true for another woman, aged 38, who had a history of serious illness and operations, including a hysterectomy and a thyroidectomy:

> *. . . or if it gets on my throat I go to the doctor and get an antibiotic . . . I don't know why, but I think with having that done I'm more conscious if my throat gets sore.*

ORGANIZATIONAL FACTORS WHICH INFLUENCE THE DEMAND FOR PHARMACY CARE

The decision to seek health care will only result in a consultation if there is adequate access to the services which provide that care. There are currently just over 30,000 registered pharmacists practising in Great Britain. The majority, around 21,000, work in community practice, either in the small chains or multiples, or independents (i.e. single pharmacies). Of the remainder around 5000 work in hospitals. The rest work in health authorities, industry, and the agricultural or veterinary sectors (1994 data). There are just over 10,000 community pharmacies in England and Wales, out of which 480 million prescription items were dispensed in 1993. According to Department of Health statistics, there was, in 1991, on average one pharmacy for every 4850 people in England and Wales (RPSGB and the DoH 1992). Distribution is very uneven however, with clusters in London and other metropolitan locations and under-provision in some areas (National Audit Office 1992). Despite variations in distribution, access to pharmacies does not appear to be problematic. A study in 1981 on access to primary care services reported that 90 per cent of those surveyed said it was very or fairly easy to get to a pharmacy (Ritchie *et al.* 1981). It has been pointed out, however, that the distribution of community pharmacies may not reflect patient needs, even though proximity to a pharmacy tends to be greater in more deprived areas (Hirschfield *et al.* 1994).

Convenience factors, such as proximity to home, doctor's surgery, child's school, work, or other shops, appear to be the most important factors determining choice of one pharmacy over another (Smith 1990a; Jepson *et al.* 1991; McElnay *et al.* 1993; RPSGB 1996). But in the context of pharmacies being used as an alternative to the GP, general practice supply factors, that is the manner in which the GP service is offered, appear to impact on pharmacy consultation rates. Easy accessibility, relating to quicker access, especially in view of the lack of an appointment system in community pharmacies, are factors cited by pharmacy clients as reasons for going to the pharmacy instead of the doctor (Ritchie *et al.* 1981; Smith 1990a; McElnay and Dickson 1994; Bissell *et al.* 1996; Hassell *et al.* 1996). Linked to this organizational issue is the financial disincentive to seeking advice from the GP. One woman from the 'Pathways to Care' study mentioned that she does not receive sick pay if she takes time off work to see the doctor. Thus, if she cannot get a doctor's appointment outside work hours she will visit the pharmacy instead.

Service-related factors become relevant to the public where a choice of convenient pharmacies exist, or where convenience is not important to people. Friendly and helpful staff (Jepson *et al.* 1991; Vallis *et al.* 1997); approachability, interest and concern shown by the pharmacist (Smith 1990a); staff knowledge; an efficient and prompt service and short waiting times for the prescription dispensing service (Povey *et al.* 1990; Jepson and Strickland-Hodge 1993; McElnay *et al.* 1993; Vallis *et al.* 1997), as well as a well-stocked/wide product range (Jepson *et al.* 1991), have all been identified as important factors in determining choice of pharmacy. The friendly and helpful service from staff also encourages loyalty to one pharmacy (Jepson *et al.* 1991).

The layout of pharmacies and the lack of privacy in them is thought to explain the low level of demand for pharmacy advice on health-related issues (Smith 1990a). The dispensary in most pharmacies is cut off from the rest of the pharmacy, giving the impression that the pharmacist is unavailable to consult, while the lack of a private consulting room precludes discussion of potentially embarrassing topics (Smith 1990a; Jepson *et al.* 1991; Vallis *et al.* 1997).

With few exceptions (Bissell *et al.* 1996; Hibbert and Elliott 1996), little research has been conducted on whether the public distinguish between multiples and independents and the sort of service they look for from each. Evidence suggests that members of the public value small local pharmacies, where customers are known to staff, for responding best to their individual needs, while the anonymized service perceived in supermarket pharmacies is not rated. Anonymity was not rated as an important reason for visiting a pharmacy in another study which explored patronage issues with customers of independent pharmacies (Smith 1990a).

Evidence from the pathways study suggests that individuals seek a different type of service from the different types of pharmacies. Local independent pharmacies are seen as a vital community resource, with customers using them because the staff are trusted, and they have a well-established relationship with them:

> . . . *I think the pharmacy has a great role to play. Say in an estate like this, I think people would go to him first for little minor things, but if it's serious you would go to the doctor, but I think they have a great role to play. They have a standing in the community and a great place for them, and I do not like them closing.*

This is made more evident when comparisons are drawn between these and the larger chains:

> *Interviewer:* So do you think they're different from the big
> chain or supermarket ones?
>
> *Respondent:* Oh yes, because they are local and for the community and the people get to know them. But there again, Boots have a fast efficient service. I am quite taken by Boots, you know. They are very, very good, and obviously they must pay more so they employ good people and they are always ready with advice.

THE IMPORTANCE OF 'PLACE' IN DEMAND AND USE OF COMMUNITY PHARMACY

There is some indication that demand for pharmacy services and the nature and quality of advice provided by pharmacies is shaped by locality (Mukerjee and Blane 1990; Rogers *et al.* forthcoming), although analysis of these differences in the pharmacy literature has been fairly superficial (Fisher *et al.* 1991). Analysis of observational data from the first of our pharmacy studies suggests that differences in the environment within which pharmacies are located and organized influence the type of service provided to local populations, such that an inverse care law may be operating in relation to the nature of services in poor urban localities compared to those in rural areas (Rogers *et al.* forthcoming). Aspects of the inverse care law relate not so much to the fact that disadvantaged groups make less use of pharmacies (though this is evident in relation to the purchasing of OTC medications), or to the accessibility of the service, but to the quality of the service and the attention people receive, and particularly to the environment within which these services are delivered. Moreover, the nature and quality of advice giving are also influenced by the internal environment of the pharmacy. This is not just related to the lack of privacy in pharmacies, but also to the manner in which the internal spacial arrangements mimic or reflect the nature of the external environment (Rogers *et al.* forthcoming). The following is a description from field notes of the location of one of the inner city pharmacies in our pharmacy observation study:

> . . . there is a high razored fence around the whole of the building which is within the health centre compound. There are metal shutters on all the glass windows and door and iron bars at the high windows . . . There are no nearby shops . . . the housing looks almost brand new but the area looks as though it is under siege. The shops are all boarded up or have grilles on the windows and doors. Large Alsatian dogs are barking through the pub fence. The shops are a pub, an insurance office, two grocers, sandwich shop and the rest are boarded up.

In an area of high unemployment, high levels of deprivation generally, and high crime levels, clients here demanded no more from the pharmacy than a basic prescription dispensing service. According to pharmacy staff only two to four people each day paid for their prescriptions. Proximity to the health centre and the low income of the local people meant that the vast majority used their GP as their first resource for any health-related problem, minor or serious, so that demand for minor ailment or other health-related advice from pharmacy staff was almost completely absent in this pharmacy. The fortress-like external features of the pharmacy were also reflected inside the store:

> *There is a small waiting area when you enter. There is a floor to ceiling [bullet-proof] glass partition between the staff and the customers which is totally enclosed apart from a small hatch at eye level. Because of the layout of the place it is very difficult to see the clients in the waiting area. This is because the glass partition has shelves full of products on it. The glass partition extends from the floor to the ceiling.*

Contrast this with the description of a pharmacy located in a similarly deprived area, but one in a small town, inside a busy shopping centre:

> *The pharmacy is located in a busy shopping centre in the centre of a small town. It is sandwiched between a shoe shop and a building society. Within 20 metres there are two large well known multiple pharmacies. There are approximately 25 shops in the shopping centre as a whole – so to have three chemists very near together means that competition is stiff. Despite this, the pharmacy is extremely busy as it seems to do a roaring trade in cut price toiletries, many people buying several items at a time . . . There are always a lot of people browsing in the shop which has a very open arrangement. The shopping centre gives out free supermarket-type trolleys and some customers bring those into the shop.*

Customers here acted, and were dealt with, as customers. Non-health activities and the purchase of non-medicinal products predominated. In this regard the social disorganization of the inner city contrasted with the organization of the smaller town, which had a more stable and mature community. While there were differences and similarities in the two pharmacies located in poor areas the biggest differences were between these two and the pharmacies in the rural locations. The following is a description of one of the rural pharmacies:

> *The shop is an extremely small room, holding about four customers at one time. The dispensary is very tiny and a long thin*

*shape. There is a little passage between the actual shop and the
dispensary area. The pharmacist cannot see the shop area from
where she sits.*

In this pharmacy the nature and context of interaction between
staff and customers was longer, more informal and the use made of
the pharmacy as a health and social resource greater. The pharmacy
was better resourced and the service more individually tailored to
the requirements of individuals. In the following incident in which
the customer explicitly states he does not want the inconvenience of
visiting the GP, the dialogue goes on for some time and ends on a
personal note about a non-health matter:

Man:	*Have you anything for that? [Shows damaged hand]*
Counter Assistant:	*Have you burned it?*
Man:	*I can't remember burning it.*
[Counter assistant to pharmacist]:	*Have you got a minute [Pharmacist's first name]?*
Pharmacist:	*Put your hand out straight.*
Man:	*The cuts seem to be moving about.*
Pharmacist:	*It may be eczema. I have got the HC cream, Fucidin H, but I would go to the doctor's with that.*
Man:	*I would do if you could walk straight in.*
Pharmacist:	*Have you been mixing chemicals?*
Man:	*No.*
Pharmacist:	*Have you used fibreglass?*
Man:	*No. I've always used Lux soap and then I went on to Imperial Leather. Do you think I'm allergic to it?*
Pharmacist:	*Hmm. Is it painful?*
Man:	*It is if it's put in cold water. Will TCP help?*
Pharmacist:	*No not really. The HC45 says not to use it on broken skin [looking at pack] and it is, isn't it?*
Counter assistant:	*You'd better call at the doctor's.*
Man:	*Oh, well I want some plasters, 35 assorted ones.*
Counter assistant:	*Right, £2.05 please.*
Pharmacist:	*What year is your Jaguar?*
Man:	*It's 35 years old.*

OTHER INFLUENCES ON DEMAND FOR PHARMACY SERVICES

TV and other advertising is likely to be a major influence on demand for pharmacy services. A marked characteristic of the nature of the public's use of pharmacies is that the OTC service, for most, appears to be very much consumer-led. In one study of 45 pharmacies in Scotland, 44 per cent of people presenting with cystitis requested a named product, while 13 per cent requested advice as well as a named product (Burke *et al.* 1992). Hardisty (1982), in an earlier study, observed that 84 per cent of all medicines were demanded outright by customers, and only 15 per cent recommended by pharmacy staff. Similar figures (86 per cent) relating to cough, cold and allergy products have been reported by pharmacists in Canada (Taylor and Stuveges 1992). The pharmacy observation study also noted the marked presence of what we termed the 'determined purchaser'. These customers, while influenced by previous use of products and previous experience of the ailment, also appeared to be influenced by advertisements they or friends and family had seen extolling the virtues of particular remedies. This encouraged them to ask their pharmacists for drugs by name, and in some cases meant that customers became hostile when faced with questions by pharmacy staff to determine the appropriateness of the purchase.

Uncertainty of diagnosis is likely to create or generate a level of demand, such that individuals will try one OTC product to treat symptoms, then go on to something else if illness remains. Masking serious complaints and delaying other vital treatment in this way is one of the major concerns about self-medication. However, little research has been conducted to explore the appropriateness of much self-medication.

How much is demand for pharmacy services shaped by GPs themselves as opposed to the way their service is structured? Recent research suggests that GPs are encouraging their patients to self-medicate (Walker 1997), either in order to save their own general practices resources or to help patients who would otherwise pay more for a prescription. There is some evidence from our pathways study to indicate that this does happen. One woman mentioned she goes to the chemist when her GP advises her to buy a cheaper OTC product:

> *The other doctors will sort of say, well you could get this and this but buy it over the counter because it's cheaper.*

However, the evidence is by no means unequivocal (Sutters and Nathan 1993; Erwin *et al.* 1997). Others have found a reluctance on the part of GPs to recommend that their patients obtain pharmacy advice because of a fear that serious illness will be overlooked. Moreover, GPs, pharmacists and consumer bodies have criticized the quality of advice given by pharmacists (Goodburn *et al.* 1991; Anderson and Alexander 1993; Consumers' Association 1994). Thus, studies which examine pharmacists' abilities to perform the advisory role and studies which explore the outcome of consumer behaviour as a result of pharmacists' advice would serve to clarify the contribution of pharmacy in primary care.

SUMMARY

This chapter has focused attention on one specific section of primary health care. In an era when GPs are keen to reduce inappropriate demand for their services, a shift of the treatment of minor ailments to pharmacy care may be appropriate. While a variety of influences are operating to encourage this movement, others work to prevent it. Supply factors encourage the use of pharmacies: long waiting times for a GP appointment, long waiting times once in the surgery, and the lack of an appointment system in community pharmacies are factors which encourage pharmacy use. However, lay beliefs about the inadequacy of self-medication products and perceptions about the legitimacy of pharmacists' role as advice givers encourage the public to continue to use general practice. The actual nature of the illnesses which are presented in pharmacies (i.e. self-limiting, recurring and minor) also limits the extent to which individuals *need* pharmacy advice. Sufferers are informed enough about the illness and know what they want to purchase, based on previous experience or other competing sources of information. The cost of prescriptions and OTC medicines and the economic resources individuals have for them interact with these influences, producing a complex set of factors which affect patients' decisions to use pharmacy care.

The pharmacy profession, in an attempt to re-establish a role for itself in the primary health care sector, has focused on issues relating to the accessibility and convenience of the service in contrast to the appointment-based service in operation in general practice. Research evidence indicates that consumers' decisions to consult a pharmacist for primary care are made, to a small extent, in the context of public awareness about the need to ration use of an over-stretched GP service. Arguably, patterns of pharmacy use are determined more by the perspective that consumers have of the professional boundaries between GPs and community pharmacists, in which pharmacists are viewed negatively, or indifferently, in terms of their diagnostic and therapeutic skills. If demand in primary care is to be better managed, with more care channelled towards pharmacy, it is possible that a shift in consumer understanding and expectations about pharmacists' expertise will be needed before larger numbers of the public begin to utilize the pharmacy as 'the first port of call'.

8

INFORMATION AND LAY
DECISION MAKING

Patients who have access to health information are better educated and
empowered to participate in their own health decisions and, as a result, will
make shared decisions that reduce unnecessary and inappropriate utilisation (thus) saving money

(McEachern)

INTRODUCTION

The nature of access to, and provision of, information is an important factor to consider in relation to the demand for and use of services. Information has come to be associated with a means of both
inducing and reducing service demand. Information supplied to
patients is relevant at the point at which they seek formal health
care. It is also relevant more generally to lay decision making within
formal health care systems and it might also play a role in the effective management of illness. Recent evidence suggests that in primary care patients' expected benefits from information in the form
of explanation and discussion of symptoms outweighs the antici-
pated benefit from the prescribing of drugs or seeing a specialist in
the secondary care sector (Woloshynowych *et al.* 1998). However,
providing information is not a panacea. Information provision and
use need to be seen in the context of patient perceptions. The
relationship between professionally provided information and its
understanding and use by patients is crucial. Moreover, relevant
information is not limited to that provided by the NHS or from
other official sources such as the British Medical Association or
Health Education Authority. People draw on other types of information which may be more influential than that from official
sources. At times the latter may have relatively little impact or

relevance in shaping people's health care actions. Information sources in late modern societies are numerous and diverse, and the plethora of information about health and illness is both positive and negative, orthodox and alternative. The Internet, which already provides some people with large amounts of interactive information about their emotional and physical health will increase access to information substantially when the Internet is made available to people through their televisions. Information from official sources designed to change behaviour or inform patients needs to be viewed against this wider background.

In this chapter we examine three aspects of information which have relevance to the decisions that people make about utilizing health care. The first section examines the relationship between information and decision making within health care generally. The second section examines critically the growth and relevance of self-care material and information provided about the use of contemporary primary care services. The last section examines the way in which 'unofficial' information provided via the mass media and 'word of mouth' might impact on lay health action around self-care and primary care more generally.

INFORMATION AND PATIENT DECISION MAKING

Patients' desire for information is not necessarily synonymous with their wanting to be involved in health care decision making (Entwistle *et al.* forthcoming). However, comprehensive information provided from official health sources has been viewed as essential to involving patients in making informed decisions about, and being active participants in, health care (Coulter 1997). An illustration of how a lack of information might relate to delays in seeking help is provided in a study by Bleeker and colleagues (1995). People with a myocardial infarction who failed to access care quickly in an emergency were found to lack appropriate information about signs and symptoms. Positive outcomes identified in a number of studies about providing information to patients include a reduction in emotional distress and anxiety when undergoing health procedures; a source of social support in promoting a patient's sense of control of his or her own illness (Dennis 1990; Paraskevaidis *et al.* 1993; Lynch 1994), and assistance in making similar decisions to clinicians placed in the same position (Mackillop *et al.* 1989).[1]

Even though there is evidence that many patients want more participation in decisions about their treatment, deficiencies in both the form and content of available patient information are reported by studies of patients. In particular there is a failure to share information about the risks and benefits of treatment. Health professionals may not provide the degree of information required by patients for their personal risk assessment and management (Rogers *et al.* 1993; Chapple 1995; Koning *et al.* 1995).[2]

BARRIERS TO THE ASSIMILATION AND USE OF INFORMATION

There are a number of barriers to the assimilation and use of information by patients.

Patient factors

Health care literature refers to memory, motivation, deficiencies in knowledge about the body, a lack of ability and confidence to make decisions, and failure to act appropriately on information provided. Studies often present researchers' interpretations of patients' motivations rather than those of the patient. For instance, one study refers to 'patients' poor knowledge about the body and its functions, together with a poor motivation for receiving "unpleasant information" '. However, this type of literature rarely takes account of the subjective meanings, actions and contexts of those being researched or of the context within which patients make decisions.

One factor in the willingness of patients to be involved in decisions about their health care seems to be related to the messages and expectations people receive about their legitimacy in being involved in decision making. As Entwistle *et al.* (forthcoming) point out:

> There are several reasons why people may be reluctant to get involved in decisions about their health care. Firstly people might not know they can play an active role in medical decision making and might not expect to do so. Cultural and professional norms in the UK have tended to reinforce the expectation that when lay people consult a health professional, they will adopt a passive role in decision making and respect the professional's judgement.

Timing and context

The timing and context of the provision of information can have an impact on its effectiveness. This is illustrated by an Australian study of the self-management of asthma (Gibson *et al.* 1995). It indicated that there are clear points at which information will be useful in decision making and other points when it is likely to be ineffective. Two groups of patients, one recruited from within a primary care context (from community pharmacies) and the other a hospitalized group, both expressed strong preferences for information concerning their condition. However, subjects preferred not to make decisions alone about the management of asthma exacerbations. As the severity of the asthma episode increased, the desire to make decisions decreased. The authors concluded that 'while asthmatics have strong desires to be informed about their illness, they do not wish to be the prime decision makers during an exacerbation'.

Professional and 'communication' factors

Health professionals' 'communication' skills have been seen as contributing to fear in patients undergoing major treatment (Jarman 1995) and some health information has been found to be incomprehensible to lay people (Dukes and Helsing 1992). The collation of information has not always taken into account the specific needs of different population groups (Ludwick 1992; Miller and Hart 1995)[3] and poor communication between doctor and patient is a frequently quoted reason for the failure of information to have the desired impact. While the notion of evidence-based decision making is growing in salience, the results of research on the effectiveness of therapies compiled in a systematic manner are generally targeted at physicians in the decision-making process. Information packages are designed for professionals not patients. Moreover, when information is provided to patients it is often of an inferior nature to that provided to health professionals. It has been found to contain factual errors, some of the advice is impractical and hazardous and it contains little epidemiological, clinical or preventative advice.

There are limitations to the assumption that professionals should have the primary responsibility for giving information to patients. These relate to the different interests and roles that professionals have in delivering care. There appear to be problems of confusion and *ad hoc* practices in information provision in general practice,

community and hospital settings (Bolton and Britain 1994). Providing information may also be viewed as a substitute for recognizing patient autonomy and allowing fuller patient participation in
decision making and care. A study which examined the perceptions
of health education practices in acute settings (Latter *et al.* 1992)
found that patient education and information giving were occurring
on more wards and more frequently than 'encouraging patients and
their families to participate in care'. The role of professionals as
providers of comprehensive and empowering health information
may also clash with their perceived responsibilities as decision
makers. For example, one study found that physicians altered their
recommendations about treatment according to how informed
patients were, suggesting a professional vested interest in controlling the nature and type of information provision (Rochaix 1989).

The potentially incongruous relationship between the giving of
information and making of decisions was identified in a study
examining women's decisions about whether or not to take hormone replacement therapy. Health professionals tended to want
minor side effects listed only if they occurred quite frequently. By
contrast, lay people wanted all effects listed, no matter how rare or
minor they were. One solution to these tensions is to separate off
the tasks of information giving from the person delivering or
responsible for health care. In the US patient education co-ordina-
tors and community-based telephone information and referral services are used to ensure that patients receive sufficient and clear
information.

The transmission of information

Another important factor related to the failure of information to
impact on patient decision making is the effectiveness of the mode
of transmission. Printed information is commonly accepted as the
simplest and most effective means of providing information to lay
people. The provision of adequately written educational material is
deemed essential to reduce patient dissatisfaction and encourage
active participation of patients in their own care (Vahabi and Ferris
1995).

Personalized educational material is considered more effective in
enhancing health knowledge than non-personalized information.
In relation to the latter, for example, videotaped information about
colon cancer was found to have more success than the use of
printed information (Meade *et al.* 1994). There is also a recognition

of the need for information to be given more than once. The way in which information is framed has also been viewed as being important in improving its effectiveness, though this does not appear to be independent of the level of risk and type of decision made (Marteau 1989). One study from the United States suggests that new technology is important in affecting attitudes and feelings of mastery towards self-care measures. Another study compared users of a computer program designed to enhance self-care for colds and 'flu with non-users. Compared with users, non-users preferred personal contact with their physicians and felt that computerized health assessments would be limited in vocabulary and range of current medical information. Non-users were also more likely to agree that people could not be trusted to do an accurate computerized health assessment and the average person was too computer illiterate to use computers for self-care (Reis and Wrestler 1994).

THE USE OF INFORMATION IN RESOLVING HEALTH PROBLEMS IN PRIMARY CARE

In the 'Pathways to Care' study, information in making decisions and resolving health care problems was mentioned by a number of respondents. Information can lead people to be proactive in formulating needs and managing illness better. In some cases it was clear that, had a range of options or information been made available from primary care at an earlier point, patients would have been in a better position to have made a decision about the appropriate form of health care. This is illustrated by the account from this woman in her 60s who sought to move on the management of her problem:

> *I suffered a lot, as I said, from my early 30s, and it's about 10 years ago that I was suffering with my back I presume and I saw this advert on television and it was just a big advert for the pain clinic at Liverpool that anyone could go to . . . so I quickly wrote it down and asked [GP] was there any such pain clinic in my neighbourhood . . .*

There was an expectation that the GP should have offered this information sooner rather than the person finding out by chance:

> *. . . the GPs do know about it, they don't look surprised when you mention the pain clinic, but they don't offer it.*

The failure to offer information in this instance was linked to a belief that the GP was being protectionist about his professional power and felt threatened by information about a service that was available from another source. In another instance, the failure to provide adequate information was an important factor for this woman who wanted to take control of her illness but felt dissatisfied and confused by the pessimistic and fatalistic view of the long-term management of her health problem and those of her family. A lack of information at different points in her contact with the GP was felt to be disempowering and inappropriate:

> ... *they don't explain, I mean I've been for brain scans and things lately, because I kept getting a lot of headaches, now the headaches seem to have gone, yes, but I've had another letter from the doctor; he, the consultant, wants to see me again, but I get a dry mouth all the time, and it's just like, oh oh, and that's it nothing to be done about it ... but they don't really discuss it with you, you know what I mean. I think that they should inform you more. I mean I've had this scan; if the scan's fine why do they want to see my brain again?*

However, even though this patient was dissatisfied with the lack of information there was a reticence about obtaining more information:

> *Respondent:* But they want to see me again to have another scan.
> *Interviewer:* Were you worried about that then?
> *Respondent:* Yeah, because I thought, well, them CT scan things, they are dear aren't they, to use on people? So they wouldn't willy-nilly test me again if everything's all right would they?
> *Interviewer:* So have you not thought about getting in touch with the hospital or ringing your doctor up?
> *Respondent:* No [laughs]. I just moan to myself.

Another woman's search for information was also linked to her desire to manage her arthritis and that of her partner more effectively herself and she was disappointed that the doctor was unable to give her more help in identifying alternative management strategies:

> *I do think he's a good doctor and he seems nice and all this, but sometimes I can't see there's nothing I can do. Like with arthritis I thought, there's got to be something, cod liver oil or something*

you do for arthritis, you hear, I don't know people with arthritis but I've heard about it and I think surely there is something. Because my husband's father he had a bit of arthritis. I'm sure he used to do something with his diet before he died.

This woman then went on to explain how, subsequently and independently of her GP, she tried homeopathic medicine and cod liver oil and got information from books:

I just thought what I've got to do now is just get a book of what you can do to prevent it getting worse.

The extent to which patients will use information in part depends on how health professionals view, promote and respond to the need for information from patients. In the next section we focus on the use by patients of information designed to affect decision making at the point of entry into the health care system.

THE USE OF INFORMATION IN MANAGING DEMAND

The public provision of information has been recognized as an important demand management tool in the US (Pencheon 1996). In the first part of this section we explore the way in which self-care manuals have been used and assessed as a demand management strategy. A nascent demand management strategy for primary care, based on providing information about self-care and the responsible use of services, has surfaced recently in the UK. We examine and raise questions about the type of information which has been provided to the public.

Self-care manuals and their impact on service utilization: the US experience

A systematic source of advice and information has been provided by self-care manuals. These have been most extensively used in the US. Written detailed material provided by health maintenance organizations (HMOs) focuses on individual decisions in the area of self-care, medical service utilization and healthy lifestyles. Reference books include, for example, 'clinical algorithms' for more than 100 problems common in adults (Vickery *et al.* 1988).

There is a disparate range of studies which have attempted to assess the effectiveness of self-care booklets. Positive results are reported in relation to the subjective acceptance and use of self-care books (Pencheon 1996).[4] There are other studies which have addressed the impact of written self-care material on service utilization. However, deductions about the extent and way in which the service use is affected are complex and ambiguous. A review undertaken some time ago reported a reduction in primary care consultations of between 7 per cent and 31 per cent in five out of seven studies. In the remaining two studies there were actually increases in the visits made to services. All of the studies concluded that there was no harm to patients from practising self-care (Anderson *et al.* 1980). In an American context a recent study of the introduction and use of a self-care manual to members of an HMO showed that four months after its introduction there had been a drop in clinic visits of 21 per cent among a group of patients who had received the manual compared with an 8 per cent drop in attendance among those who had not (Elsenhans *et al.* 1995). However, the researchers of the first randomized controlled study of a self-care approach concluded that, on its own, a comprehensive self-care manual did not have proven efficacy as a demand management strategy:

> A self-care book that guides patients in seeking home care or physician care for 63 medical problems was assessed in three randomly selected groups of families to determine the book's effect on the number of visits to physicians. The first group was given the book and an optimal seminar on its use; the second group was identical to the first but each family was promised $50 if their visits to physicians dropped by one third; the third group was a control group. The book had no significant effect on the number of physician visits during six and 12 month study periods, even though one half of the families read most or all of the book, and more than one third used it for a specific medical problem. Large-scale distribution of this self-care book therefore did not result in significantly less dependence on physicians for treatment of acute medical problems.

According to the researchers, the lack of proven effectiveness is not surprising. In a debate with the authors of the self-care manual used in the trial (who interpreted the same findings in a more positive light) they stated:

> The literature on changing well-established behaviour patterns is replete with studies that show how difficult it is to effect even

a small (10 per cent) change in behaviour. Therefore it is not surprising that simply distributing a self-care book and offering a seminar (which was poorly attended) and financial incentive will not decrease physician visits by 21 per cent or greater. For our talk with book recipients, it will require more intensive efforts such as triage persons at the physician's office or group educational sessions to change the way they use the medical provision system when all care is paid for.

(LoGerfo *et al.* 1981)

More encouraging results were reported by a subsequent random-ized controlled trial (RCT) of a similar self-care manual. This reported a statistically significant decrease of 15 per cent in total medical visits for a Medicare population compared to a control group (Vickery *et al.* 1988). However, a number of issues suggest that evidence for the success of even comprehensive and detailed self-care booklets is still equivocal, in so far as their impact on utilization of services is concerned, and is unlikely to be simply generalizable to the UK context. First, the decreases in service use are quite modest when seen in the cultural context of heavy mar-keting and the generation of demand for health care services by health care providers in the US. Second, methodological questions about the sample size and type of households used in RCTs like the one above (which enrolled 1,009 families) suggest a need for caution in interpreting the magnitude of impact on utilization rates.[5] Self-care booklets targeted at specific conditions (such as back pain) and evaluated in a British context have suggested the likelihood of only a modest impact on rates of utilization (Roland and Dixon 1989). Third, self-care booklets may not, in certain cir-cumstances, reduce the 'right' sort of demand, and may even delay the appropriate use of services. For example, in the Vickery *et al.* study (1988), the reduction in health care use for minor ailments was found to be not significantly different between the control and experimental group. In another study, which examined the use of self-care booklets by mothers dealing with childhood ailments, the authors concluded that despite significant benefits, the mothers in receipt of the self-care booklet intervention were more prone to rely on self-care even when the need for medical care was indi-cated. This may suggest a reliance on self-care when it is at odds with professional advice (Rasmussen 1989). Finally, the effective-ness of self-care booklets may be time-limited (Cherkin *et al.* 1996),[6] and the processes which lead people to reduce utilization following receipt of a booklet remain something of a black box. Given the complexity of findings about the impact on utilization from a range of different studies, a systematic review of the existing evidence about the impact of self-care manuals on health care utilization is required to clarify further the benefits and limitations of such strategies. In-depth qualitative research built into the design of RCTs may also do more to illuminate the processes of change in the beliefs and actions of people who are the subjects of such interventions.

Combining the use of information with other strategies

Other self-care strategies have also been evaluated for their effectiveness and used as alternatives or as supplements to an informational approach. One approach has been the development of self-care programmes involving behavioural techniques used to target key groups, such as those suffering from anxiety, tension or stress. For example patients presenting with medically unexplained physical symptoms (MUPS) can be treated effectively with cognitive behavioural therapy (CBT)[7] (Speckens *et al.* 1995). While such techniques have been found to be effective, they remain labour-intensive and time-consuming, and are likely to be suitable for development in relation to specific groups of patients only. A further danger is that such programmes, by focusing on individual capacities for change, may act to mask social and economic inequalities which result in high rates of anxiety and stress (McLean and Peitroni 1990).

More recently, and building on previous self-care manuals, a further development in the US has been to combine the use of self-care with triage and other health services management systems. A combination of streamlining authorized referrals and information is being used as a demand management tool in HMOs, with encouraging preliminary results. The basis of this approach is the establishment of 'call centres'. In these, a computerized clinical information system combines medical triage expertise and patient-specific information as the basis of managing demand for services. The system is run by nurses using a structured line of questioning and discovery which replicates the thinking of a GP in diagnosing and dealing with a problem. A highly specific range of self-care measures is used. Reportedly for some HMOs this service experiment has been so successful that primary care physicians have been concerned about being bypassed completely (Morissey 1997).

However, a more equivocal note is struck in a recent report, which suggested that the 'results of studies on telephone triage are about equally split between those that show no significant change in demand and those that show reductions' (CSR5 Report 1997). 'NHS Direct' the new advice line introduced as part of recent NHS reforms is modelled on HMO's telephone service.

Information on self-care and the responsible use of services: the UK experience

An 'NHS 50th birthday' self-care manual has recently been distributed by the Department of Health and written information about self-care has also been used in localities in the UK, though far less extensively than in the US. One example is the primary care out of hours co-operative in Greenwich, which has used literature on self-care as a resource for managing health problems. This written material (called 'What should I do? Do I go to the doctor?') was implemented in four localities in Greenwich and Bexley Health Authority in May 1996. A preliminary evaluation found that 95 per cent of local GPs wanted patients to have self-care information, and so did 90 per cent of a sample of 2000 patients who were interviewed prior to the introduction. The 'Doctor/Patient Partnership'[8], however, seemingly represents the first national public campaign aimed at the management of demand. The aims of the campaign, launched in 1996 were described in a press release from the British Medical Association (BMA):

> The 'Doctor/Patient Partnership' was launched jointly by the Secretary of State for Health and the Chairman of the Medical Services Committee (GMSC) in February 1996 to encourage the appropriate use of NHS general medical services by publicising out-of-hours initiatives and educating the public to use GP services properly.

In the absence of a formal evaluation of the scheme it is not known whether, and in what way, the dissemination of information about self-care and use of services has changed patient views, attitudes or behaviour, in terms of accessing services or self-care measures. Analysing some of the campaign material does however highlight some of the dilemmas and difficulties in getting across consistent and appropriately targeted messages. Explicitness of purpose and consistency of messages are likely to be minimum criteria by which to judge the quality of information. In this regard it seems a number

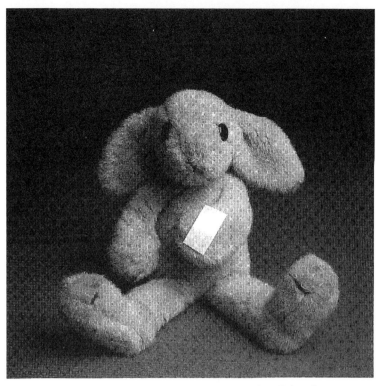

ENJOYING EASTER

Puffers, pills and plasters

Don't run out over Easter.

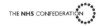

Figure 8.1 BMA bunny

of pertinent questions need to be posed about the likely effectiveness of presentation and content.

What, for example, are we to interpret from the use of a bunny
rabbit to convey messages about encouraging aspects of self-care
and using services responsibly? The 'It's Cool to Cover Up' campaign, for example, 'uses a picture of the cuddly bunny mascot clad
in sun hat, T-shirt and sunglasses' (*Pulse News*, 7 June 1997). The
same bunny reappears in a subsequent 'Get Ready for Coughs and
Sneezes' campaign in which the 'BMA bunny has taken to bed with
a handkerchief and a self-administered dose of paracetamol' (*BMA
News Review*, 24 September 1997). There is a tradition in Britain of
using cute animals to convey health and safety messages to children. (Tufty the squirrel was used to promote road safety messages
in the 1960s, for example.) But the target audience of the BMA
campaign are on the whole adults, not infants. The mascot image
clashes with the notion of independent adults taking responsibility
for their health, and it might provoke hostility in well-informed
patients, who may feel patronized.

A second question relates to the clarity and logicality of the message. The information combines two separate issues – self-care and
the responsible use of services. Consequently there is an ambiguity
about how the preventative self-care messages – e.g. covering up
from the sun or uptake of childhood immunization – fit with the
responsible use of services. Other health information sources and
interpretations of the nature of illness are also important factors to
consider. For example, in the September campaign, the symptoms
of the common cold and 'flu are described as being 'coughs and
sneezes'. But does such a description accurately apply to influenza?
Is it always a minor ailment, benign and self-limiting, like the
common cold? To what extent can the apparent symptoms of 'flu be
distinguished from more serious respiratory infections such as
pneumonia? To highlight the ambiguity we raise here, there are two
conflicting official lines of information being disseminated about
influenza. One is about self-care aimed at *reducing* service utilization and the need for professional consultation. Another is about
inducing service contact (for vaccination) via messages that virulent
viruses are on the increase and even life-threatening (implying the
need for professional surveillance and expert treatment).

Perhaps the greatest confusion relates to using services responsibly and appropriately. What, for example, does that mean in the
absence of comprehensive and widely available information about
when and what services are available? Are patients universally
informed about opening hours and availability of services?

Moreover, if GPs are not to treat minor ailments, then what is their role in the provision of health care? The Doctor/Patient Partnership initiative has recently been joined by a parallel information campaign run by the Royal College of General Practitioners. They have produced a series of leaflets: *How to Work with your Doctor*. Separate leaflets deal with: *How the Family Doctor Service Works*; *You and your GP During the Day*; *You and your GP at Night and at Weekends*, *Coping with Minor Ailments*; and *Getting the Most from your Pharmacist*. They provide specific advice on each of these areas. The form and content of service provision, particularly out-of-hours services, vary significantly and it is therefore unlikely that even well-researched[9] campaigns like the RCGP initiative will be able to provide detailed enough information about service availability which will cover the diversity and idiosyncratic nature of primary care provision which operates in specific localities. It is likely that NHS Direct which will have computer access 'to multiple sources of services[9] in a locality will be of more' assistance to people seeking care for a specific service.

More generally there has been a significant development of the amount and diversity of official information provided to the public. Many health care funders and providers now produce leaflets and advertisements to persuade people to adopt particular patterns of health care use (see Box 8.1). Few of these campaigns have been rigorously evaluated and people are exposed to many competing and inconsistent messages from diverse sources. Unofficial sources of information about health are also likely to be important in the way in which patients make decisions about using services and in undertaking self- and alternative health care activities.

THE RELEVANCE AND USE OF UNOFFICIAL
SOURCES OF KNOWLEDGE ABOUT HEALTH
AND ILLNESS

In addition to official information, 'unofficial' sources of information from a variety of sources are important in shaping people's actions and knowledge about health care and expectations about service provision. They also feed indirectly into the formulation of demand for primary care services. The media, friends and relatives are sometimes the main source of information about therapy and provide an important supplement to information provided by professionals. One recent study, for example, found that out of 490 women who had consulted their GP for vaginal symptoms, 65 per

---

Box 8.1 Examples of information materials intended to influence self-care and consultations in primary care in the UK

When Should I Call the Doctor? Getting the Most from your Local GP Services
This leaflet was produced by North Yorkshire Health Authority and distributed to all households. It covers various common health problems, giving suggestions for self-care and indicating which symptoms warrant contacting a doctor or the emergency services. It tries to discourage use of 'out-of-hours' services for non-urgent problems without dissuading people from contacting their doctors in 'real emergencies'.

How to Work with your Doctor
The Royal College of General Practitioners led the production of this series of leaflets which contains five titles: *How the Family Doctor Service Works*; *You and your GP During the Day*; *You and your GP at Night and at Weekends*; *Coping with Minor Ailments*; and *Getting the Most from your Pharmacist*. The leaflets aim 'to help people understand how the family doctor service works and enable them to get the best health care from their general practitioner'.

Heavy Periods? You Can Get Help
A leaflet produced by Buckinghamshire Health Authority and other local agencies and groups. It stresses that heavy menstrual periods are a common problem and that there are treatments that can help (hormonal and non-hormonal drugs, and surgical options). It encourages women with heavy periods to discuss the problem and the treatment options with their doctor.

---

cent informed themselves further from encyclopaedias, leaflets and women's magazines, and 68 per cent discussed their symptoms with partners, families or friends (O'Dowd *et al.* 1996).

The media is an important source of information about health and illness which has relevance to the use of primary care services, the way in which individuals assess their own health and undertake

Box 8.2 Sources of health information that may influence self-care and help-seeking behaviours

- Family, friends, work colleagues, acquaintances
- Community leaders, local people recognized as sources of health-related advice
- Self-help groups and voluntary organizations
- Consumer health information and advice services e.g. telephone help lines, high street and hospital information points
- Health food retailers
- High street pharmacists
- Health care providers outside the 'official' health care system e.g. acupuncturists, chiropractors, herbalists, homeopaths, osteopaths, spiritual healers
- Health care providers within the 'official' health care system e.g. dentists, doctors, health care assistants, homeopaths, nurses, occupational therapists, physiotherapists
- Individuals associated with health care providers e.g. relatives/friends of health professionals, medical receptionists
- Pharmaceutical companies
- 'The media' e.g. news items, specialist health features, advice columns or programmes, health-related episodes in dramas and soap operas.

self-management strategies or seek alternative forms of care. The media has been viewed as a mediator of medical messages, values, definitions and concerns to the lay public, and is seen as providing an opportunity for lay people to express their views while simultaneously altering them (Karpf 1988; Gabe *et al.* 1991). The reporting of health problems can also impact on patient action (Anderson and Larson 1995). Popular books, newspapers or lay magazines may influence both lay and professional providers of care. New ideas and suggestions about acceptable and controversial treatments have been found to reach the lay person before the professional and to act as a source of information via lay people to professionals. These informal sources impact both on the expectations about services and the way in which people use other means and responses to health care problems using self-care or alternatives. Data from the 'Pathways to Care' study illustrate these points.

INFORMATION AND ITS IMPACT ON EXPECTATIONS ABOUT SERVICES

Information about health services is available to large numbers of people in the population through a variety of media and from local knowledge; these are important in shaping people's expectations about services. Coverage of the NHS often focuses on the costs, shortages and pressures faced by the NHS and these were frequently alluded to by the respondents in the 'Pathways to Care' study. The use of services for patients in our study took place against a background of the perceived pressures the NHS and primary care were working under. This frequently included the mention of rationing and a limited supply of welfare and public services more generally. Background information about the pressures of the NHS at times coalesced with information and experience picked up locally, for example the experience most people had of short consultation times, or the perception that GPs had no time to listen because they had too many patients to see and were working under constant pressure. This elderly man, who consulted and was undergoing tests for a suspected vascular problem in his leg, was an example of someone with limited expectations about services:

> *Interviewer:* *Did you have any expectations of what might happen at the consultation?*
>
> *Respondent:* *No. I've learnt not to. Yeah, I mean, I've learned there's nothing, not everything is as it should be like. I've got no complaints about it [the health centre], erm, like everything else it's become limited. Well, limited in that because of an increase in population, whereas, erm if we've got fewer people attending that there is far greater time able to be allocated to the individual whereas if you've got more people then time has to be allocated to everybody and as a result there will be a degree of difficulty on behalf of the staff there to be able to do that.*

The man had also come to hear of plans to increase the size of the surgery:

Well that [development] is in the pipeline, because they've got to saturation point and like everything else, it gets overfull and you have to look at how they are fulfilling their obligation. As far as the GP is concerned I would say that the same also applies, in that, erm, C as a town is increasing and also the constraints put on them by the bureaucrats means that a lot of that time that they could allocate to patient care is being sort of absorbed. There is greater strain being put on them [GPs].

Although this man reported being personally unaffected by such change, *'because I know what I want to see him about so I don't sort of deviate from that'*, this did suggest a message about the need to be quite straight and to the point about the reason for consultation, so as to fit in with an under-resourced and over-burdened system. A number of people reported that the GP did not have time to listen to them. If this does in fact characterize consultations, then complex problems which cannot easily be dealt with may result in an unsatisfactory meeting on need and attendance. There were, for example, two instances where the intended consultation for one problem (depression, and anxiety about a suspected heart problem) were substituted when contact was made with the doctor for the presentation of another problem (a cold which was clearing up, questions about medication for a stroke).

SOURCES AND USE OF 'UNOFFICIAL' INFORMATION ABOUT HEALTH PROBLEMS AND TREATMENT

In the 'Pathways to Care' study, people only infrequently reported not wanting or using information from whichever source it came but it was clear from some people's accounts that not everyone wanted more information than they were presently given. One elderly middle-class woman reported never reading newspapers or other items about health. She went out of her way to avoid reading about health promotion thought that the media exaggerated all health risks, and did not want to be informed about any health matter by her GP:

One of the doctors at the office tried to give me a nice informative chat one day about thrombosis and, err, something else, aneurysm, I think it was, and I said, 'Look,' I said, 'don't tell me anymore, I don't want to know, I live on my own', I said, 'and

> *I'm not going to sit up in bed at night counting lipids in my blood. I don't want to know. Ignorance is bliss'.*

Similarly, this elderly couple responded in the following way to a question about whether they had been aware of any health campaigns on the television or in the press: *'No, don't bother, they've been on but we ignore them'.*

Elderly respondents seemed to make less use of information, mainly because they saw it having less relevance to them, as indicated by this 75-year-old woman:

> *Interviewer: And what do you think about women's magazines on how they cover health issues?*
> *Respondent: I don't read them.*
> *Interviewer: Do you not look at them at all?*
> *Respondent: No I never read them, I can't be bothered with them. Too old for that.*

Most people however thought that information of all types and from a variety of sources was useful[10] and there was evidence of an eclectic use of information from different sources in managing everyday health problems. For example, one woman who was interviewed reported using old-fashioned remedies such as lemon tea and whisky for colds which her mother had taught her about. When her husband developed diabetes, she went straight to the library and got books on the subject. She used camomile tea for sleeping, having read about it in a magazine, and used a herbal remedy called 'Natracalm' which she had seen advertised in a health food shop. The use of herbal remedies or supplements, such as garlic tablets and primrose oil, were most frequently learned about from kin, friends or magazines, rather than from official sources such as the health centre or health education leaflets.

The influence and processes related to the use of information differed for different people. Three types of use of information were identifiable from the accounts in the 'Pathway to Care' study. The second type of user was most common:

- Some people consulted medical books, or read items in magazines but did not act on these sources of information, relying instead on authorized information from the doctor.
- Some people used information as a supplement to information and advice provided by the doctor or after formal health care failed.

• Some people had a preference for using information as an alternative to going to the doctor.

Three households reported using a multiplicity of alternative therapies instead of accessing the GP. Rather than going to the GP one man preferred to try herbal remedies for colds, used primrose tea for its calming effect and Tiger Balm for his arthritic knee and for headaches. He had tried Alexander technique and had been to see a homeopathic doctor. He had also taken Ginseng, Kelp and garlic tablets. He took arrowroot for constipation and when he had 'flu he boiled up lemons with sugar and water.

Written information was used by people in a variety of ways. Information from informal sources acted as a means of accessing official knowledge at the point of identifying a problem. A woman with breast cancer went to the GP when she had a wart that changed colour. She had seen something about it on the TV. It acted as a form of therapy as well as information: *'Magazines give you a bit of inside information of how to cope a bit more.'* Other people in the study also reported turning to information provided in books as a means of support, especially when formal sources were seen to have failed. When one woman was told that nothing could be done for her arthritis she turned to a book to see how she could prevent it from getting worse. One woman who found that her doctor's help was not effective for her irritable bowel syndrome went to classes and bought a book which helped. The solutions from alternative sources were at times seen as less invasive than allopathic medicines, for example: *'it's just that I didn't want to keep trying different medicines'* – the medicines made her feel worse so she used a book to find out information about how to change her diet.

Information from magazines and elsewhere also acted as a check on the knowledge and actions taken by health professionals and indirectly provided a resource for negotiating and managing a response from the health care system. (It seems that magazines and other sources may for most of the time be the only source of evidence-based medicine available to the public.) At times alternative sources of information were even viewed as life-saving. Here an elderly woman reports such an incident to the interviewer:

> *Respondent: One of the ladies I go out to see she diagnoses everything from a magazine and she's very good actually. I mean she's been very poorly and she's had lot of things and she's diagnosed everything.*

> *Interviewer:* I was going to say, What do you think about women's magazines?
> *Respondent:* I think they must be very good because she's been spot on and I think she's saved her own life.
> *Interviewer:* Really?
> *Respondent:* Yeah by telling the doctor different things. Yeah, because she was on Warfarin and, err, they really got it wrong, they gave her far too much and her blood was thinning out like nobody's business, she was coming up in bruises all over.'

There was also one example of how information broadcast during an epilepsy week helped provide a resolution to a serious behavioural problem in a child of seven:

> *We have problems with the eldest who is seven, but recently we found out some more information. I was epileptic and when I was pregnant with him I was on epileptic drugs. And it was all by accident, err, my Mum had read it in the* Radio Times. *I came round Thursday morning from shopping, put the tele on in the ktichen and blow me they had an epilepsy help line number on. It's always something that niggled me and I think it's something called Foetal Anti-Convulsion Syndrome. It's, erm, they have behavioural problems, speech problems, eyes, they have all sorts of problems. I rang up the line. I rang this woman and I was explaining about J about how he was and she said, 'How does he sleep?' and I said, 'Well he goes to bed he's fine but then he's up and down four or five times, "My arm, my leg, this hurts here", and I say, 'Go to bed, it's only growing pains' [laughs], she said it could be true. So I said, 'Why?' 'Well,' she said 'when you were pregnant the Epanutin drains the Vitamin D out of your body.' I mean I was going through a pint and a half of milk a day, 3–4lb of cheese a week and bananas something terrible and she said, 'Yeah'.*

When she received the written information pack she went back to discuss the new information with the GP who was reported to have been receptive:

> *I'd booked the appointment for J and I went in and he said, 'Oh you've come with an envelope but where is the child?' I said, 'He's in the envelope' [laughs]. Now he's been very good, he's referring us back [to the specialist] and he would like to know more about it . . . We got what we want.*

This account provides an example of how lay people can sometimes become more knowledgable and active about a problem they are invested in than the GP and also about the potential utility of advice lines and information that are available outside of the formal health service. In this instance the professionals seemed willing to 'learn' from the mother's knowledge and the outcome was positive, despite ambiguity over the long-term prognosis of the problem: *'the school are interested, our doctors are interested, the speech therapist is interested and the occupational therapist is interested'.*

Information backed up by health expertise or other knowledge about health carried considerable weight. One man reported discussing how he found out about remedies from the person who had taught Alexander technique at a class he had attended. In another instance the presence of a qualified health expert in a kinship network had the effect of limiting the authority to give health advice to others in the same network:

> *Interviewer: Do you give your family any [health] advice?*
> *Respondent: I don't really need to. Because I'll tell you I'm well connected, my second daughter is a nurse.*

Another example was provided by an elderly women who reported not using magazines or leaflets about health matters but instead drew on her training as a PE teacher in devising her own self-care strategies:

> *It goes back a long way. I was trained to teach PE. And when I was trained, as well as being trained to do PE we did massage, with me doing gymnastics. So I was training to be a physio, erm, and masseur as well. So I had got a lot of knowledge. I know how my body works if you like.*

SUMMARY

This chapter has focused on three aspects of the relevance of information in managing demand. First, the culture and factors affecting the way in which patients make decisions about health care. Second, the use of self-care manuals and triage systems in the US, and recent public campaigns about self-care and patient responsibility which have emerged recently in Britain. The third and final aspect concerned the role played by unofficial sources of knowledge in everyday health care practices. The discussion of the complex effect that each of these has on shaping the use of services and impacting on patient behaviour suggests that simplistic approaches to the development and dissemination of information are likely to result in little change among population groups. While it was evident from our study that a number of respondents wanted more information, it is worth noting here that not only are people exposed to many competing and often inconsistent messages from diverse sources, but people vary in the way they interpret information about health care (Frewer *et al.* 1994). This is because they attach different meanings to language and symbols and understand illness within different conceptual frameworks and belief systems. Perceptions of the credibility of information may also be affected by the extent to which it fits with prior experiences of illness and health care and by opinions about the information producers.

The results about the effectiveness of self-care manuals are promising but equivocal. In particular, the processes behind changes in the use of services remain unclear. Additionally, given the apparent success of sophisticated triage systems in the US, it seems likely that information strategies, together with changes in the configuration of and access to services, are likely to be more effective in managing demand, better at least, than a reliance on written self-care material alone or special pleading to use services more responsibly. An informational approach will also, it seems, need to tackle the conceptions, presumptions and roles of professionals in involving patients in health care decisions. Finally, the knowledge and information that patients have about alternative ways of dealing with problems might usefully form the basis of information to professionals who may be unaware of health care strategies that patients find useful and could be more widely incorporated into advice giving to other patients.

The challenge of a future agenda in ascertaining the role that information on health and illness might have on patient actions is to develop methodologies which are able to tap the complexities of assessing the ways in which patients make use of information from a variety of sources and how they make sense of competing wisdoms inherent in different types of knowledge.

NOTES

1 For example, in a hypothetical study about consenting to participate in clinical trials about cancer treatment, lay consent was compared to that

of clinicians (Mackillop *et al.* 1989). Clinicians were found to be far less likely to consent to treatment than the lay 'surrogates'. Subsequently, respondents were told about the decisions which doctors would make in the same circumstances and asked if this information would modify their previous decision. The proportion of people consenting to the chemotherapy trial decreased by 40 per cent.

2 Chapple (1995), for example, notes the inadequacy of current practice in relation to providing information to patients about hysterectomy. Patients have also identified a lack of information in relation to mental health treatments, side effects and alternatives (Rogers *et al.* 1993). In the area of respiratory care, unmet needs identified during research have been associated with the need for information about diagnostic tests, prognosis and long-term use of medication.

3 In a study of the information provided about breast cancer, for example, both the lay and professional literatures were found to have inadequately addressed the degree of risk and the special needs of elderly women (Ludwick 1992). A failure to target key groups has also been a concern of commentators evaluating the HIV/AIDS health education literature (Miller and Hart 1995).

4 For example 'Healthwise' (a self-care initiative) used by a number of HMOs has shown that 73 per cent of participants in a self-care programme consulted with their handbook and 59 per cent consulted their handbook/telephone system prior to calling the doctor.

5 Moore *et al.* above, for example, had previously entered into a debate with Vickery *et al.* about disputing the conclusions that can be drawn from differences between control and experimental groups in a previous RCT using a book devised by Vickery and colleagues and had stated: 'We calculated that future studies will need nearly 2,500 families to reliably detect a true 7.5 per cent reduction because of the book's effect if population with similar variability in use are studied' (LoGerfo *et al.* 1981).

6 A randomized controlled trial of a patient education intervention for back pain conducted in the US suggests the time-limited effectiveness of professionally communicated educational material. Three groups received different packages. One group was given a 15-minute face-to-face consultation with a nurse together with a telephone follow-up, a second group was provided with an information booklet and the third group received 'usual care'. Though patients in the nurse intervention group reported greater satisfaction, the researchers reported that differences in self-perceived knowledge and self-reported exercise were no longer significant after seven weeks. There were also no significant differences among the three groups in worry, symptoms, functional status, or health care use at any follow-up interval (Cherkin *et al.* 1996).

7 CBT works on the basis of a practitioner engaging with people's own self-defeating cognitions as a means of working together to solve a problem.

8 Despite the title of the campaign which suggests an input from patients or their representatives, patient involvement in the campaign was absent. The origins of the campaign emerged as part of the conciliatory package surrounding the negotiation of the terms of the GP contract as part of the settlement about the remuneration of out-of-hours working. The campaign has been greeted enthusiastically by the professional medical press but with reservations by consumer organizations. The patients' association criticized the first campaign, which was about not calling the GP out unnecessarily, claiming that older patients would be frightened to contact their GP and would suffer in silence.

9 Preparing the leaflets involved research to find out what was already available, a large number of organizations were consulted and the leaflets were piloted with both doctors and patients.

10 46 out of the 55 interviewed reported using some self-care or advice from elsewhere.

CONCLUSION: MANAGING DEMAND BETTER AT THE INTERFACE BETWEEN LAY AND PRIMARY CARE

... the pressures on the NHS are exaggerated. Indeed they have always been exaggerated ... Rising public expectations should be channelled into shaping services to make them more responsive to the needs and preferences of the people who use them.

A modern and dependable national health service will capture developments in modern medicine and information technology. It will build around the needs of people, not of institutions and it will provide prompt reliable care.

(Department of Health, *The New NHS: Modern Dependable*)

INTRODUCTION

During the course of this book we have focused on a number of arenas relevant to understanding the formulation of demand. From an analysis of a wide-ranging literature and our own research we have shown the diversity and complexity of the relationship between need, demand and use of services at the interface between lay people and formal primary care.

In Chapter 1 it was shown that definitions of health need and its relationship to demand are contested and reflect underlying tensions and interests. Within the NHS approaches to the problem of demand have tended to focus on changing 'supply'. This supply focus emphasizes the reduction of ineffective treatments and rationing existing services resources. Patient factors, and in particular the 'rising' public expectations about what health care services can provide, have also been seen as a factor contributing to rising demand. However, such a concern has not traditionally been linked to an in-depth consideration of the way in which people, express need, formulate demand, use services and make decisions about managing illness. The failure to link supply with demand means that the interaction of professional and organizational factors have been separated from the needs and actions of those accessing and using the health service. In Chapter 2, we saw that a thinly veiled culture of blaming the patient for 'inappropriate' demand in primary care has emerged in some quarters. There are particular complaints about the use or 'abuse' of out of hours services by patients. Again, this has been without reference to the evidence which points to the role of GP action and organizational arrangements in generating and shaping demand or to the fact that hitherto out of hours services have been considered to be an intricate part of primary care services. Changing assumptions about this commitment and new arrangements for out of hours primary care contact (e.g. co-operatives) have generally been made without reference to public views and expectations.

In Chapter 3, we concluded that from within the world of health services research traditional approaches to understanding utilization have generally preferred to separate out and weigh independent from dependent variables as a means of identifying the factors responsible for utilization rates. However, as we saw in later chapters, not only are dependent and independent variables not easily separated out in this way, but such an approach fails to capture the diversity and complexity of influences on pathways to care. The social process model has illustrated the importance of the process of seeking care and the meaning of actions taken by ordinary people in accessing care. When the in-depth action of patients in using services and managing illness are viewed as being grounded in their personal experience, everyday lives and immediate social contexts, then a different picture emerges of the factors influencing the use of services. As we have seen in Chapters 4–8, the experience of illness is shaped by a number of inextricably linked processes and factors. These relate to personal experience, aspects of identity, biography and social position, social networks and access to diverse sources of health knowledge and information. Within the lay arena, responses to illness are in constant flux, according to changes in the condition and everyday contingencies. The responses reflect both the way health situations are assessed and the resources available at the time to manage illness. Our own research illuminates aspects of the link between locality and lay health action in using formal primary care. In Chapter 4 this was evident in the way in which people viewed the causes of illness. In Chapter 7 our analysis pointed to differences in the nature and quality of advice and services provided by pharmacies operating in disparate localities which is likely to impact on the type and quality of resources that people have access to prior to, or instead of, contacting formal primary care services.

In Chapters 6 and 7 we explored the roles of social networks in influencing health action and providing informal care. The latter are helpful in some circumstances in providing advice and care, and influencing the point at which contact is made with services. However, with some problems advice may be readily provided but other problems are more difficult to deal with. For example, it is difficult both to seek and find ready advice for psychological problems. The influence of lay networks also varies considerably between individuals and according to personal health biographies. In this regard the demand for informal care is, like formal health care, subject to limited resources and is 'rationed'. This implicates a continued need to respond to inequalities systemically and in a way which transcends the divide between lay and formal provision of care. A lack of social and community resources in dealing with health problems outside the health service reinforces the need to concentrate resources in promoting access to formal health provision and developing services which meet the needs of disadvantaged groups. Chapter 4 also illuminated an important relationship between supply and demand. The experience of having used services in the past is a significant influence on subsequent demand and help seeking. People learn over time how to fit into what is required of them by professionals when using the health service. This may engender less confidence about using self-care measures or trying alternatives. Negative experiences of health care may induce a reluctance to use services again, resulting in health needs remaining unmet. Conversely it may encourage consultation in an attempt to gain needed help, reassurance or problem resolution for illness which might have been managed more appropriately initially.

What was also clear from both the literature and patient accounts in our own study was the coalescence of a range of disparate influences, beliefs and knowledges on help seeking. People's reported actions in the pathways to care study contained reference to both their immediate social context and contacts with others in the use of primary care and other parts of the NHS as well as 'alternative' ideas about health and illness gleaned from a range of different sources. (For example, the health experiences of relatives living abroad was a dominant influence in two of our interviews.) At times accounts of people's health actions appeared to be fragmentary and contradictory. (For example, one or two interviews contained accounts of assessing and evaluating symptoms and attempts at self-care in one illness episode, which sat alongside descriptions of apparently less serious episodes of illness in which a person sought help from the GP.) Distinctive patterns of help-seeking or self-care practices were thus difficult to identify and are equally difficult to suggest a uniform health 'policy' response to. There were none the less points at which the importance of the reaction from primary care to health problems did take on a particular type of salience. The point at which the nature of a particular health problem is uncertain or worrying for patients is one example where primary care professional/patient interaction seems to take on a heightened significance and where the availability of information and alternative choices of management appeared to be particularly important to patients. Similarly, and confirming other sociological research, those who were further along illness careers often seemed to expect less from primary care and seemed to have firmer views about where the boundaries should be between self- or lay management of illness and the seeking of formal health care. (This was particularly evident in relation to mothers who had children suffering from asthma and those with musculoskeletal problems such as arthritis.)

Turning to the conclusions from Chapters 7 and 8, both community pharmacy and information initiatives have an important potential in both mediating and managing demand. While there are a number of supply factors operating within formal primary care that point to the untapped potential of community pharmacy to play an increasing role in managing minor and self-limiting ailments presently seen in general practice, there are number of barriers that may prevent this occurring. This includes a questioning from lay people of the perceived efficacy of medications and appropriateness and acceptability of the advice available from community pharmacy and a more general questioning of the legitimacy of the pharmacists' role to extend to areas which have traditionally been dealt with by GPs. In Chapter 8 we saw the important but ambiguous and multivarious role played by information in influencing use of services. This implied the need for a systematic appraisal of the impact that different types and sources of information are likely to have on people's health care actions and decision making.

A POLICY AND PRACTICE RESPONSE TO MANAGING DEMAND

The illumination of the complexity and diversity of the influences on the formulation of demand suggests the need for a reappraisal of the policy and practice response to managing demand. The use and demand for services reflects a process in which it is not possible meaningfully to separate factors such as individual knowledge and response to health and social situations from the need for and use of services. Given the inextricable link between the contact with primary care services[1] and the way in which people use services the analyses we have presented here suggest the need to overcome the separation between needs assessment activities on the one hand and service response on the other. In terms of an evidence-based research, development and policy agenda this implicates the need for a shift in emphasis from *analysing* need and demand to *developing strategies* for dealing with it effectively. This would need to take into account the importance of the influences outlined here (i.e. people's assessments of and experience of illness and service use, social and network resources, the use of lay, self- and alternative sources of care and health knowledge). Managing demand more effectively in primary care is likely to require a policy response which takes cognisance of:

- the diversity and complexity of health action among different groups in the population and points in the illness career,
- access as an interaction between organizational factors operating in primary care and people's health and social resources and perceptions of services,
- the diversity of information sources and means by which it is utilized within the health service and delivered to the public,
- exploiting the possibilities of providing responsive care based on a combination of lay/informal and professionally provided care.

Implicit to the existing range of mechanisms for dealing with demand are a number of strategies which might be developed in a direction which more effectively manages demand at the interface between lay and primary care. We consider here the ones most likely to have an impact at this interface in the near future.

CHANGING HEALTH BEHAVIOUR IN ORDER TO
CHANGE SERVICE UTILIZATION

It may be remembered from Chapter 1 that modifying the health and illness behaviour of population groups has been a prominent strand of thinking in the area of demand management. The most successful attempts to modify or change behaviour can be seen in health promotion strategies and interventions which take as their starting point patients' perceptions, resources and actions. In the area of health promotion, recent AIDS campaigns have tended to work with and build on people's own definition of the problem and their own behavioural strategies to protect their sexual health. Less success has been achieved in areas where lay resources and environmental constraints provide less scope for changing behaviour. This has led at times to a victim blaming approach to the issue, as with smoking among working-class mothers (Graham 1987). A different direction is evident in very recent public health policy. This seeks to make a link between the structural determinants of health and health behaviour and effectively influence health status and preventing ill health by developing health promotion as part of main stream primary care services (e.g. 'healthy living centres') interlinked with other key health and social welfare organizations and policy initiatives (Department of Health 1998).

At the level of modifying illness behaviour evidence-based practice can also be applied to provide practical solutions to altering the pattern of illness behaviour and service use of 'frequent attenders'. As we discussed in the previous chapter, behavioural interventions targeted at some groups of frequent and 'inappropriate' attenders have been shown to be effective. However, there are some cautions about this enthusiasm for the applicability of therapeutic solutions to complex problems (apart from the problems of applying successful interventions undertaken in an experimental situation to everyday primary care practice). Therapeutic solutions are only applicable to a small number of people in the population. Even though a small number of patients may make frequent use of services, rising demand has a variety of other causes. Conflating rising demand with a small sub-population of intensive utilizers tends to pathologize the wish or need to use health care on the part of the whole population. Thus, while such targeted behavioural interventions might be part of the solution, they are likely to be only a part. A systemic approach which responds to the wider context and processes implicated in the generation of demand is also required. The development of new and imaginative responses within primary care which transcend the informal/formal care divide by drawing on and resourcing voluntary and 'alternative' approaches to self-care might also supplement the individualistic response of behavioural interventions.

INFORMATION ON SELF-CARE AND SERVICES

Targeted information about self-care and the availability of services has an important role to play in demand management. Information about the effectiveness of health care is required to allow people better access to knowledge in making decisions about the management of their own health. Offering people more meaningful information is one way of giving people some control over the process of managing illness and seeking help appropriately. Sophisticated self-care material and interactive information, such as videotapes from surgeries and the internet could be increasingly exploited. Though the need for information which is targeted, effective, appropriate and acceptable to different groups in the population is well established, to date this is an under-developed area which presents particular challenges to which policy makers need to respond. Few information campaigns have been rigorously evaluated, and people are exposed to competing and often inconsistent messages from diverse sources, and vary in the way in which they interpret information about health care. Additionally, perceptions about the credibility of information will be affected by prior experience of illness and by opinions about the information producers. A crude policy of 'let them have information' is unlikely to be successful in isolation from other measures. Information alone, however well it is produced, is likely to have only a modest impact on help-seeking behaviour. Thus a strategy for producing and disseminating more meaningful and targeted information needs to be integrated with other forms of health support and changes in service provision.

GRADUATED ACCESS

Our pathways to care study suggested that 'access' to care is usefully viewed as an interaction between organizational factors operating in primary care combined with people's perceptions of services and individual social circumstances in seeking care. One way of modifying demand and responding to need differently is to change the nature of service provision at the point at which people want to access services. By international standards the low cost of British primary care, together with its open access, is enviable. However, the present configuration of services is not necessarily the most effective or appropriate. As we have seen, out-of-hours visits are a particular point of tension. People are increasingly being given messages that they must not call out the doctor 'inappropriately' and are being made to feel increasingly guilty about the use of such services. At the same time, doctors are seeking ways of reducing their commitment to providing out-of-hours care as a way of reducing their overall workload. They have concerns about their increased and increasing tasks and duties and the length of their working day. One response to this has been to change the pattern of care provided through the establishment of GP co-operatives and primary care emergency centres, which provide greater levels of telephone advice than more traditional services. However, in general the most notable feature about the current arrangements is the lack of a graduated service or the comprehensive ability to respond to health problems. There is a role for integrating self-care actions combined with the exploitation of new technology and other sources of advice and information. For example, there is a need for ordinary parenting action to be supported and improved by accessible advice and telephone support. The next level of access might be a visit to an out-of-hours centre. Further gradations of access could be created to offer a service which is more responsive to the particular needs of patients. Such a strategy would need to be sensitive to the differential resources people have in using health care. For example, people who do not have ready access to transport to make a visit out of hours may still need a visit at home or transportation provided in order for them to access services. Responding to financial resources and increasing access by removing barriers at the level of community pharmacy is important for some patients. For example, for those who cannot afford to pay for an OTC product, a GP consultation is a means of accessing a free version of a similar one. Greater and more conspicuous out-of-hours access to pharmacists and advice lines may also be a useful means of opening up another resource to assist self-care activities.

Both the need for information and graduated access implicate the scope for greater use of 'direct health services'. Direct health services are ones which the public can access without having face-to-face contact with professionals and which maximize the use of new technologies. They encompass the use of telephone systems, automated or supported by expert triage systems; video links (e.g. telemedicine); direct mail services (e.g. direct access to pharmaceuticals and diagnostic devices); Internet services; view text services; or cable television. These types of services have been used successfully elsewhere, particularly in managed health care systems in the US (Robinson and Steiner 1997). Consideration is also being given to how these may be adapted and incorporated in the UK.

Opening up other direct access points and encouraging the development of mutual support and self-help groups, which are easily accessible (e.g. based in primary care buildings), could also provide an alternative source of care and advice, forming part of a system of graduated access crossing the boundaries between informal and formal health care sectors. This might form part of the commissioning and providing strategy for primary care groups and local health improvement programmes outlined in the recent White Paper. If they are to be effective, graduated levels of access need to be based on models of service that are sensitive to the particular needs and conditions of patients and incorporate an acknowledgement that people's use of services are shaped over time rather than instantaneously.

PERSON-CENTRED PRACTICE

Changes in access arrangements are likely to be of most use in managing discrete episodes of illness. However, as we have seen, an 'episodic' view of health and illness is limited in so far as it does not deal with the ongoing use of health services or management of health problems which more accurately reflects the reality of people's experience of illness. An over-reliance on direct services might also result in new forms of unequal access for those groups in the population who do not have the resources to or are unaccustomed to dealing with health matters in this way (e.g. elderly people). It has been noted that such services are likely to exacerbate existing disadvantages in access to services for black and ethnic minority groups if responding to specific linguistic needs are not inbuilt (Free and McKee 1998).

Additionally, direct services will not (and many would argue should not) replace the personal contact that most people have come to expect from the NHS. A positive relationship and good communication between primary health care professionals and patients are not only a matter of the quality of service provided at a point in time. Contact with services and the quality of consultations with health professionals also influence the *subsequent* way in which people manage their health and illness. Chapters 5 and 6 focused on the importance of the personal experience of illness in shaping our responses to managing illness. There is an inextricable link between the past experience of illness, use of services, personal identity, and the immediacy and impact of social context on help seeking. Contact with professionals is a relevant component in this complex process. This indicates the desirability of promoting a greater responsiveness to the individual expression of illness by the health service. 'High-trust' relationships would be fostered by a culture of shared control between patient and professional providers. With greater patient–professional congruence would come a mutual sharing of control, risk, responsibility, information and decision making. Changes currently taking place within primary care and medical education which emphasize a problem-based approach to learning and the promotion of alternative models of consultation style and content are relevant here. Components of patient-centred practice provide one model which might promote such a patient–professional partnership and is presently in common currency within some primary care practice in the UK (May and Mead in press). This comprises six defined professional attitudes/ values identified by Stewart *et al.* (1995):

- Exploring the disease and illness experience – there would be an openness to patient-presented problems, a receptiveness to patients' cues, feelings and fears, and responsibility for non-medical aspects of problems. Sensitivity to unconscious or hidden motivations for seeking help might also be involved.
- Understanding the whole person – this entails a respect for the patient's uniqueness and autonomy, and an acceptance of diverse personal and cultural backgrounds.
- Finding common ground regarding management – this entails a willingness to collaborate and share management responsibility with patients. It respects the patient's values, preferences and expressed needs. It enables patients to make informed decisions.
- Incorporating prevention and health promotion – this values health promotion and invests time and energy in incorporating screening and prevention in patient care.
- Enhancing the patient–doctor relationship – this accepts the risk

of exposing weaknesses and uncertainties. The doctor is prepared to act as the patient's advocate.

- Being realistic – this involves professionals being aware of their
own limitations and personal responses to stress. They are willing
to ask for help when it is needed.

Professional–patient relationships based on these principles are
likely to help break the pattern of medical paternalism and passive
patient relationship as the basis for establishing mutual and shared
understandings and responsibilities in managing illness.

THE HEALTH SERVICE–PATIENT PARTNERSHIP
IN MANAGING DEMAND EFFECTIVELY

A different understanding of the public, and the way in which they
use health services, will need to underpin a changing culture within
the NHS. For example, health professionals would have to accept a
new principle of lay access to large amounts of information traditionally within the exclusive domain of health care professionals.
Access to codified health knowledge and information about services
would lead to more empowered patients which would inevitably
challenge further the basis of the existing professional–patient
relationship. Becoming aware of external influences and working in
a way which complements the social realities and health practices of
lay people and other agencies (e.g. employers) would require
changes. These would not only be at the level of interaction between
professional and patient, but would require mutual participation in
developing responses to health problems that crossed the boundaries between social, health and lay provided care and resources.

Similarly, a different type of response would need to develop
towards 'rising' public expectations about what health care services
can provide. As we have discussed at various points in this book,
this is often construed as patients wanting or demanding more
under conditions of increased rights and limited responsibility.
These 'expectations' have been responded to by restricting and
rationing services as a way of preventing use. However, such a strategy is likely to be counter-productive since perceived scarcity of
services may inadvertently drive up the need to use services (Pencheon 1998). Conversely, free and open access may be more likely
to tap into people's existing 'responsibilities' and assumptions
about access to the health services. A different response to the

attempts of user campaigns to achieve greater responsibility and control over health and health care is also implicated. Such campaigns have frequently encountered barriers of professional interests and professionals have been reluctant at times to concede power and autonomy.

The principles of partnership, mutual risk sharing and control point to the need for greater involvement of ordinary people more generally in primary care. There is a history of involving users in primary care from which lessons might also be drawn in the contemporary era. An early example of this is provided by the Peckham experiment, credited with a revolutionary approach to primary care. It owed its genesis to lay people.[2] It came from them and was *responded* to by professionals (Pearse and Crocker 1943). There are contemporary models of good practice in primary care which incorporate user participation in delivering primary health care though these are likely to bring with them a new set of challenges and dilemmas for primary care (Pietroni and Chase 1993). By drawing on the expertise of lay people in conjunction with developments in primary care provision, new alliances and approaches in managing demand effectively can be forged.

THE NEW NHS POLICY AGENDA AND MANAGING DEMAND BETTER

The data show that a better understanding of demand from a patient perspective has implications for managing demand differently, suggesting considerable challenges in terms of an adequate response from policy makers. In this final section we draw attention to the way in which aspects of recent government policy are likely to fit this agenda and areas where it may not. An underlying theme to the approach taken in this book has been the failure to reconstrue the policy agenda about demand management. Past and current analysis of the 'demand management' problem have tended to present a 'doomsday' scenario of what will happen if patient expectations continue to rise. Analyses of the problem have drawn on images of a demographic 'time bomb', increasing pressures on the NHS exemplified in burgeoning waiting lists and overflowing Accident and Emergency Departments. Correspondingly espoused solutions have tended to be reactive. The latter have included: 'doing nothing' based on naive assumptions about growth within available resources to 'keep things ticking over' (Øvretveit 1997;

Ham 1998); sacrificing comprehensiveness (e.g. by rationing out a number of effective (elective) treatments; sacrificing universality with social and private insurance for some and a NHS safety net for the rest; and questioning the 'free at the point of use' nature of the health services by considering the introduction of co-payments. It may be argued that these analyses carry with them a healthy degree of realism (idealism in the NHS has had a bumpy ride over the last two decades).

However, recent policy changes are likely to permit a degree of divergence from this previous approach in opening up possibilities for developing a more positive approach towards managing and responding to demand. The central tenets of *The New NHS* White Paper and the public health Green Paper *Our Healthier Nation* include :

• a recognition of the active responsibilities and roles that ordinary people play in the management of illness and their potential influence on the way in which services are used (e.g. by stressing the need for increased access to information and advice, the importance of 'fair' access in using services and the focus on tapping into patient and carers' experiences of using the health service as a barometer of the success of the service),
• a commitment to developing more responsive NHS services and maximizing communication and the provision of information using modern information technology (e.g. the provision of faster advice and information to people in their own homes via the 'NHS Direct' – the public telephone triage and help line),
• a multi-sectoral approach to responding to health need and demand which crosses health and social care boundaries.

Additionally, the proposed development of primary care groups (PCGs) and trusts bring with them the hope of greater flexibility in responding to demand through service development. Independent primary care trusts will be responsible for commissioning all primary care services with an integrated budget. The explicit aim in setting up PCGs is to attune service provision to local needs by improving the quality, range and accessibility of services, tackling unmet need and developing organizational models of health care delivery which integrate community with primary care. This agenda provides a continuum in terms of building on the opportunities offered recently by locality purchasing arrangements which have allowed primary care physicians to expand their range of services and their ability to reach out to people (Garr *et al.* 1993). Larger commissioning and provider groups are likely to permit the development of a wider and different range of services than is possible under the current arrangements for primary care. Similarly, 'NHS Direct' – the new telephone advice and information line – is an example of developments which may better fit people's experiences of using services in other sectors (e.g. 24-hour banking, video links and increasing use of the Internet). The Green Paper *Our Healthier Nation* also outlines a multi-sectoral approach to tackling unmet need and inequalities in health by offering opportunities to forge links between what is provided as part of a health service and the public, private and lay sectors. Health Action Zones are being set up to explore new, flexible and local ways of delivering services which offer a means of responding to inequalities and health need by making the connections between environmental, social and economic policy initiatives and those within the health service. Engaging and working with the aspirations of citizens and 'patient involvement activities' is likely to be given a higher profile than hitherto as it constitutes the explicit focus of the Patient Partnership R&D initiative launched in early 1998.

There is a cautionary note to add to this overall optimistic outlook. As well as opportunities there are likely to be substantial barriers to developing a patient-centred approach to demand management. The emphasis on developing commissioning in line with managed care principles are likely to provide opportunities for providing packages of care, which are informed by strategic need assessment activities. However, they may run counter to responsiveness and flexibility at the individual level. It has, for example, been suggested that the NHS cannot afford to give patients choice or be responsive to their needs for NHS commissioning to be effective (Light 1998). The new White Paper emphasizes the need for primary care groups and trusts to work with the support of health authorities in developing and implementing health needs strategies. However, there are few explicit references or proposals about working to develop new types of services involving users of services. Developing and implementing new models of care are likely to require a greater emphasis on blurring the distinction between lay and formally provided care than has been evident in recent years. The impact of local user-centred activities and more centralized initiatives such as the 'Patient Partnership R&D Strategy'[3] on the culture and development of Primary Care Group and Trust development is likely to be important. Wider acceptance of a broader definition of health outcome and evidence (e.g. process outcomes and acceptability and appropriateness of strategies to patients) inform-ing research into the effectiveness of demand management strat-egies will also be relevant to the way in which the policy agenda develops.

Finally, but importantly, there are also a plethora of professional and organizational barriers and interests which will continue to act as a brake on new developments. Access to effective medication and the provision of services in a different way; further deregu-lation of medicines; the availability of, and access to, services from different points in the system; the inclusion of self-help groups in the mainstream of services and extending activities such as pre-scribing rights to other professional groups (e.g. pharmacists and nurses); and the embracing of the use of information technology in delivering services to patients – these are just the tip of the iceberg in the need to bring about change.

NOTES

1 This is matched by the increasing complexity of professional primary care networks operating within the health service. These relate to the intricacies of working within and across the boundaries in the NHS. Changes in health and community care policies and professional prac-tices among some groups, such as community nurses, also mean that there are increasing demands to work across the health and social care boundaries.

2 This started first in 1926 as a health club and later developed into the larger pioneering centre seven years later.

3 The 'Patient Partnership and R&D Strategy' is a Department of Health initiative launched in early 1998 which explicitly supports the develop-ment of information for patients, carers and the public, and user involve-ment in service development. It is intended to complement aspects of the recent White Paper on the NHS and Green Paper on public health.

APPENDIX: METHODOLOGY

The data drawn on throughout this book are derived from studies conducted at National Primary Care Research and Development Centre (NPCRDC) (see Box A.1). While detailed information about each of the studies is available on request, brief details of the three studies are given below.

STUDY 1: 'PATHWAYS TO CARE'

Most of the exemplars used in Chapters 4–6 and 8 are derived from this study. In July 1995 the National Primary Care R&D Centre began work on a feasibility study exploring the methodological options for and feasibility of providing systematic information on:

- the characteristics and circumstances which distinguish frequent users of health care from non-users in different social groups and for different conditions,

---

Box A.1 Studies which generated data used in this book

- Study 1: *Pathways to Care* – a multi-method feasibility study exploring the nature and scale of formal and informal health care utilization, including the factors which trigger presentation to formal and informal sources of care. This involved a household survey, a diary study and in-depth interviews with individuals in three contrasting localities. Quotations from the in-depth interviews are presented in the book in italics.
- Study 2: *Observation in community pharmacy* – an observation study of advice-giving in community pharmacies.

- the external and internal factors which trigger presentation to different sources of care – formal and informal,
- the nature and scale of formal health care use in relation to different morbidity profiles.

The feasibility study comprised the following components:

- a household and health diary survey for collecting new information on primary health care use,
- follow-up qualitative interviews to explore and understand the determinants of use, and the nature and influences on decision making among key, primary care user groups.

While empirical data in the book are mostly drawn from these latter interviews, in order to provide the context within which the primary data were collected, details about the design of the main survey, the samples, and what data was collected at each stage are given below.

Design of the empirical study

A nationally representative sample was considered too costly and time-consuming for a feasibility study. Therefore, we decided to confine the survey to three areas in the North West region. Nevertheless, it was essential that the survey should cover people with different demographic, social and economic characteristics, people of varying states of health and people with different patterns of health care utilization. Hence, probability samples were selected for three very different areas which also formed the basis for the qualitative purposefully selected sample:

- a relatively deprived urban area,
- a socially mixed urban area,
- a relatively wealthy town servicing a semi-rural area.

These three areas are referred throughout the book as Br, B and C respectively.

In order to analyse the relationship between health care utilization and health status, age, sex and socio-economic characteristics it was necessary to oversample frequent users of health care services. An equal probabilities sample would not have provided enough frequent users for the analyses. Frequent users were defined as those who had had five or more contacts with the GP practice in the preceding six months. Individuals who were thought to be at risk of using health services more frequently, i.e. young children aged 0–4 and adults aged 75 and over, were also oversampled. Two methods of oversampling frequent users were tested: oversampling from medical records and a screening survey of households. The population of interest included children as well as adults. This was achieved by selecting one adult in the household to provide information about all household members. The adult who knew most about the health status of

all household members was selected as the respondent. Trained inter-
viewers from a market research company conducted face-to-face interviews.

In order to collect prospective data on health utilization, after the face-
to-face interview was completed, respondents were also asked to complete
health diaries. The most knowledgeable adult completed information daily
on all household members. Gift vouchers (£10) were given as an incentive.
Follow-up qualitative interviews were later conducted with a small sample
of respondents from each of the three areas.

A summary of the sampling strategy for the main household survey and
sample details achieved for each of the three components of the study, for
each of the three areas separately, is given in Box A.2 below. Details of
information collected in the survey, diaries and interviews are summarised
in Box A.3.[1]

The qualitative interviews, which on average lasted an hour, were conducted in people's homes. They were audiotaped, fully transcribed and are
being analysed with the help of a computing word processing package.
Recurring themes are being noted, highlighted and grouped together. In
this book we have used the qualitative interviews to provide exemplars of
key themes and topics identified in the study and to provide broad messages from our reseach about the influences and nature of help seeking and
use of primary care services. This has by necessity involved a selected use
of qualitative data to illuminate key points.[2] A systematic analysis of our
qualitative data forms the basis of articles, which are being written up for
peer reviewed journal articles.

STUDY 2: OBSERVATION IN COMMUNITY PHARMACY

This study specifically addressed the topic of advice giving within community pharmacies. Previous research had quantified the extent of the
activity in community pharmacy, and had argued that levels of advice
giving were high, especially around minor ailments. Subsequent White
Papers emphasized the contribution community pharmacy could play in
managing minor conditions, suggesting that a shift in the public's use of this
primary care service would decrease demand for GP consultations for
'trivial' conditions. Despite this, empirical research on the *nature* of advice
giving in community pharmacies and the nature of demand for community
pharmacy services was scarce. There was also little data on consumer perceptions of community pharmacy, and on whether use of community pharmacies was in any way shaped by use and views of general practitioners'
services. In this context, this particular study aimed to:

- describe the nature of advice giving in a community pharmacy context,
- explore organizational and other factors which affect the nature and type
  of advice provided,
- better understand the impact of advice giving on customers' perceptions
  and health care action, and

Box A.2 'Pathways to Care' study summary of study design

Area 1 (Br):
- a random sample of 324 eligible addresses was selected from the Postcode Address File
- a screening questionnaire was used to oversample (potential) frequent users
- 135 households responded to the screening questionnaire (response rate = 42 per cent)
- 96 screened households were included in the sample of which 95 households (246 individuals) agreed to the structured interview
- 60 households (152 individuals) completed a health diary over four consecutive weeks
- 25 in-depth interviews conducted with a sample of health diary respondents.

Area 2 (B):
- a stratified sample of 210 patients was selected from the medical records of one GP practice in the area with oversampling of (potential) frequent users (200 patients were eligible for the survey)
- the selection of an individual implied selection of his/her household
- 122 households (300 individuals) agreed to the structured interview (response rate = 61 per cent)
- 84 households (214 individuals) completed a health diary over four consecutive weeks
- 26 in-depth interviews conducted with a sample of health diary respondents.

Area 3 (C):
- a sample of 210 patients was selected from the medical records of one practice in the area (188 patients were eligible for the survey) 45–50 patients were sampled at random from each of the following groups
- (a) residents in communal establishments
  (b) people with particular chronic conditions
  (c) the elderly infirmed
  (d) remaining patients
- the selection of an individual implied selection of his/her household
- 33 residents in communal establishment and 96 households (a total of 288 individuals) agreed to the structured interview
- 71 households and communal establishment residents (a total of 183 individuals) completed a health diary over four consecutive weeks
- 14 in-depth interviews conducted with a sample of health diary respondents.

Box A.3 Data collected in the different stages of the 'Pathways to Care' study

Household survey:
Retrospective data on health status; use of health care, including general practice, other formal primary and secondary care services, and alternative health care; demographics; socio-economic information, and a section on respondent feedback. Many of the questions were taken from the *1991 Census*, the *General Household Survey*, the *Health Survey for England* and the HEA survey on *Health and Lifestyles*.

Health diaries:
Prospective data on the daily experience of symptoms and illness, self-care activities and contacts with health care professionals were recorded in a four-week structured health diary.

In-depth Interviews:
Sixty-five interviews were carried out. Interviews covered episodes of illness experienced by members of the household identified in the survey. The interviews related to households of different sizes and composition. Just over 50 per cent of households was owner-occupied with most of the remaining households rented from the local authority. Fifty per cent of households had an income of less than £10,000 a year. Most of the key respondents were women.

These interviews were conducted to find out more in-depth information about the reasons why people decided to visit their GP when they did, and how they dealt with the problem prior to visiting the GP. More specifically they were asked about the following:

- Health status
- Behaviour undertaken to stay healthy
- Nature of particular illness episodes: their causes and associations, previous experience
- Contact with other people: lay or professional
- Experiences of and attitudes towards their GP
- Experiences of and attitudes towards pharmacists and other health care professionals
- Use of and views about medicines: prescribed, OTC and alternative
- Family agendas about health
- Use of information
- Primary care policy
- Perceptions about appropriate and inappropriate demand.

- understand the role played by pharmacists in the provision of primary health care.

Study methodology

The study used a variety of techniques to answer the different research objectives. Direct observation of customer and pharmacy staff interactions was employed to explore 'real life' primary care and advisory role behaviour. One observer spent one full week in each of ten pharmacies in the North West of England, which were sampled to represent, as far as possible, the diversity of pharmacy types and locations. Pharmacist characteristics were also considered when recruiting the pharmacies. Recordings of the interactions were made manually using shorthand notes and the resulting verbatim transcripts analysed according to emerging themes and typologies.

Pharmacists were interviewed to obtain their views on their primary care and advisory role. To establish brief customer profiles, another interviewer also collected brief data from 1000 pharmacy customers on the reasons for their visit. In order to explore users' views of pharmacists' advisory role and the outcome of advice, semi-structured telephone interviews were also conducted with 44 service users who had received advice. Observations and interviews took place in the pharmacies between November 1995 and April 1996.

NOTES

1 Further details about the feasibility study are available on request from the authors.
2 We have also drawn on one or two interviews from pilot qualitative interviews which formed part of the development work undertaken to establish the NPCRDC research programme on population health need and demand. We are very grateful to Helen Busby and Gareth Williams for having undertaken some of these early interviews.

BIBLIOGRAPHY

Adamson, C. (1997). Existential and clinical uncertainty in the medical encounter: an idiographic account of an illness trajectory defined by inflammatory bowel disease and avascular necrosis. *Sociology of Health and Illness*, 19(2): 133–60.

Allsop, J. (1994). *Health Policy and the NHS*. London: Longman.

Allsop, J. and Mulcahy, L. (1996). *Regulating Medical Work: Formal and Informal Controls*. Buckingham: Open University Press.

Alonzo, A. (1980). The mobile coronary care unit and the decision to seek medical care during acute episodes of coronary artery disease. *Medical Care*, 18, 297–318.

Alonzo, A. (1984). An illness behaviour paradigm: a conceptual exploration of a situational-adaption perspective. *Social Science and Medicine*, 19, 499–510.

Anderson, C. and Alexander, A. (1993). Response to dysmenorrhoea: an assessment of pharmacists' knowledge and its application in practice. *International Journal of Pharmacy Practice*, 2, 180–3.

Anderson, J., Blue, C. and Lau, A. (1991). Women's perspectives on chronic illness: ethnicity, ideology and restructuring of life. *Social Science and Medicine*, 33(1), 101–13.

Anderson, J., Morell, D., Avery, A. and Watkins, C. (1980). Evaluation of a patient demand education manual. *British Medical Journal*, 281, 924–6.

Andersen, R. (1968). *A Behavioural Model of Families: Use of Health Services Center for Health Administration Studies*. Research Series No. 25. Chicago: Center for Health Administration Studies, University of Chicago.

Anderson, R. (1995). Revisiting the behaviour model and access to care: does it matter? *Journal of Health and Social Behaviour*, 36, 1–10.

Anderson, R. and Aday, L. A. (1978). Access to medical care in the US: realized and potential. *Medical Care*, 16(7), 533–46.

Anderson, R. and Larson, D. (1995). Reconstruction and augmentation patients' reaction to the media coverage of silicone gel-filled implants anxiety evaluated. *Psychological Reports*, 76(3), 1323–30.

Anderson, R. and Newman, J. (1973). Societal and individual determinants of medical care utilization. *Milbank Memorial Fund Quarterly*, 51, 95–124.

Anson, O., Rosenzweig, A. and Schwarzmann, P. (1993). The health of women married to men in regular army service – women who cannot afford to be ill. *Women and Health*, 20(1), 33–45.

Anthony, R., Shorrock, P. J. and Christie, M. M. (1995). *Pharmacy Based Needle and Syringe Exchange Schemes: An Evaluation Within Trent Region*. Leicester: Trent Health Authority.

Antonovsky, H., Maoz, B., Pilper, D. and Arad, T. (1989). Personal and health factors associated with frequency of visits to the primary care clinic. *Family Practice*, 6(3), 182–7.

Araya, R., Wynn, R., Leonard, R. and Lewis, G. (1994). Psychiatric morbidity in primary health care. *British Journal of Psychiatry*, 165, 530–3.

Arber, S. and Ginn, J. (1992). Class and caring – a forgotten dimension. *Sociology*, 26(4), 619–34.

Armstrong, D., Granville, T., Bailey, E. and O'Keefe, G. (1990). Doctor initiated consultations: a study of communication between general practitioners and patients about the need for reattendance. *British Journal of General Practice*, 40, 241–2.

Armstrong, D., Bird, J., Fry, J. and Armstrong, P. (1991). Perceptions of psychological problems in general practice: a comparison of general practitioners and psychiatrists. *Family Practice*, 9, 173–6.

Arne, S., Anderson, M. A. and Loake, M. (1983). A causal model for physician utilization analysis of Norwegian data. *Medical Care*, 21(3), 266–79.

Attias, J., Shemesh, Z., Bleich, A., Solomon, Z. *et al.* (1995). Psychological profile of help-seeking tinnitus patients. *Scandinavian Audiology*, 24(1), 13–18.

Audit Commission (1994). *Finding a Place*. London: Audit Commission.

Audit Commission (1996). *What the Doctor Ordered: A Study of GP Fund-holding in England and Wales*. London: HMSO.

Auslander, G. and Litwin, H. (1990). Social support networks and formal help-seeking differences between applicants to social services and non-applicants. *Journal of Gerontology*, 45(3), 112–19.

Backett, K. (1992). Taboos and excesses: lay health moralities in middle class families. *Sociology of Health and Illness*, 14(2), 255–74.

Backett, K. and Davison, C. (1995). Life course and life-style – the social and cultural location of health behaviours. *Social Science and Medicine*, 40(5), 629–38.

Baker, M. and Kirk, S. (eds) (1995). *Research and Development for the NHS: Evidence, Evaluation and Effectiveness*. Oxford: Radcliffe Medical Press.

Balint, M. (1956). *The Doctor, His Patient and the Illness*. London: Pitman.

Bankoff, E. A. (1994). Women in psychotherapy – their life circumstances and treatment needs. *Psychotherapy*, 31(4), 610–19.

Banks, M., Beresford, S., Morell, D., Walker, J. and Watkins, C. (1975). Factors influencing demand for primary medical care in women aged 20–44 years: a preliminary report. *International Journal of Epidemiology*, 4, 189.

Barker, C., Pistrang, N., Shapiro, D. and Shaw, I. (1990). Coping and help-seeking in the UK adult population. *British Journal of Clinical Psychology*, 29, 271–85.

Barofsky, I. (1978). Compliance, adherence and the therapeutic alliance: steps in the development of self-care. *Social Science and Medicine*, 12, 369.

Barsky, A. J., Wyshak, G. and Klerman, G. L. (1986). Medical and psychiatric determinants of outpatient medical utilization. *Medical Care*, 24(6), 548–60.

Barwani, S., Panton, R. P. and Morley, A. (1987). Survey of public opinion about the community pharmacist as a source of health advice. *Pharmaceutical Journal*, 239, R15.

Baving, L. and Olbrich, H. (1996). Anxiety in alcoholics. *Fortschritte der Neurologie Psychiatrie*, 64(3), 83–9.

Beck, U. (1987). Beyond status and class in V. Meja *et al.* (eds) *Modern German Sociology*. New York: Columbia University Press.

Bell, J. (1844) quoted in Holloway, S. W. F. (1991). *Royal Pharmaceutical Society of Great Britain 1841–1991: A Political and Social History*. London: Pharmaceutical Press.

Bendelow, G. (1996). A failure of modern medicine? Lay perspectives on a pain-relief clinic. In S. Williams and M. Calnan (eds) *Modern Medicine: Lay Perspectives and Experiences*. London: UCL Press.

Bendelow, G. and Williams, S. (1996). 'The end of the road'? Lay views on a pain-relief clinic. *Social Science and Medicine*, 43(7), 1127–36.

Bendtsen, P., Bjurwf, P., Trell, E., Lindstrom, F. and Larsson, J. E. (1995). Cross-sectional assessment and subgroup comparison of functional disability in patients with rheumatoid-arthritis in a Swedish health care district. *Disability and Rehabilitation*, 17(2), 84–99.

Ben-Shlomo, Y. and Chaturvedi, N. (1995). Access to health care provision in the UK: does where you live affect your chances of getting a coronary artery bypass graft? *Journal of Epidemiology and Community Health*, 49, 200–5.

Bentzen, N., Christiansen, T., Terkel, C. and Pedersen, K. M. (1989). Self care within a model for demand for medical care. *Social Science and Medicine*, 29(2), 185–93.

Berkanovic, E. and Telesky, C. (1981). Social networks, beliefs, and the decision to seek medical care: an analysis of congruent and incongruent patterns. *Medical Care*, 20(10), 1018–26.

Bevan, A. (1961). *In Place of Fear*. London: Heinemann.

Bhrolchain, C. M. S., Klein, L. and Smith, M. J. (1993). Children with disabilities and the Children Act – who will assess their needs? *Public Health*, 107(2), 101–6.

Birkel, R. C. and Repucci, N. D. (1983). Social networks, information seeking, and the utilization of services. *American Journal of Community Psychology*, 11(2), 185–205.

Bissell, P., Ward, P. R. and Noyce, P. R. (1996). *Advising the Public: A Study of the Advice-giving Function of the Community Pharmacy.* Manchester: Academic Pharmacy Practice Unit, University of Manchester.

Black, R. (1993). *Hospital Admission Rates of Patients of GPs in Deprived Areas.* Edinburgh: Information and Statistics Division, Trinity Park House.

Blane, D., Smith, G. D. and Bartley, M. (1990). Social class differences in years of potential life lost: size trends and principal causes. *British Medical Journal*, 301(6749), 429–32.

Blaxter, M. (1985). Self-definition of health status and consulting rates in primary care. *Quarterly Journal of Social Affairs*, 1(2), 131–71.

Blaxter, M. (1990). *Health and Lifestyle.* London: Tavistock/Routledge.

Blaxter, M. and Britten, N. (1996). *Lay Beliefs about Drugs and Medicines and the Implications for Community Pharmacy.* Manchester: Pharmacy Practice Reseach and Resource Centre.

Blaxter, M. and Paterson, E. (1982). *Mothers and Daughters.* London: Heinemann.

Bleeker, J. K., Lamers, L. M., Leenders, I. M., Kruyssen, D. C. *et al.* (1995). Psychological and knowledge factors related to delay of help-seeking by patients with acute myocardial infarction. *Psychotherapy and Psychomatics*, 63(3–4), 151–8.

Blenkinsop, A. and Bradley, C. (1996). Patients, society and the increase in self-medication. *British Medical Journal*, 312, 629–30.

Bloor, M. (1985). Observations of abortive illness behaviour. *Urban Life*, 14(3), 300–16.

Bloor, M. (1995). A user's guide to contrasting theories of HIV related risk behaviour. In J. Gabe (ed.) *Medicine, Health and Risk.* Oxford: Blackwell.

Blount, R. L., Bachanas, P. J., Powers, S. W. and Cotter, M. C. (1992). Training children and parents during routine immunizations. *Behaviour Therapy*, 23(4), 689–705.

BMA News Review, *Pulse*, 24 September 1997.

Bolton, V. and Britten, M. (1994). Patient information provision: its effect on patient anxiety and the role of health information services and libraries. *Health Libraries Review*, 11(2), 117–132.

Borkan, J., Reis, S., Hermoni, D. and Biderman, A. (1995). Talking about the pain: a patient-centred study of low back pain in primary care. *Social Science and Medicine*, 40(7), 977–88.

Bororsson, A. and Rastam, L. (1993). The patient's family history: a key to the physician's understanding of patients' fears. *Family Practice*, 10(2), 197–200.

Bott, E. (1971). *Family and Social Network*, 2nd edition. London: Tavistock.

Bowling, A. (1995). *Measuring Disease.* Buckingham: Open University Press.

Bradshaw, J. (1972). The concept of social need. *New Society*, 30 March.

Briscoe, M. E. (1987). Why do people go to the doctor? Sex differences in the correlates of GP consultation. *Social Science and Medicine*, 25(5), 507–13.

British Market Research Bureau Ltd. (1987). *Everyday Health Care: A Consumer Study of Self-medication in Great Britain*. London: BMRB Ltd.

Brown, C., Rowley, S. and Helms, P. (1994). Symptoms, health and illness behaviour in cystic fibrosis. *Social Science and Medicine*, 39(3), 375–9.

Brown, G. W. and Harris, T. (1978). *The Social Origins of Depression: A Study of Psychiatric Disorder in Women*. London: Tavistock.

Brown, G. W., Burley, J. and Wing, J. K. (1972). Influence of family life on the course of schizophrenic disorders: a replication. *British Journal of Psychiatry*, 121, 241–58.

Burke, P. M., Richards, R. M. E. and Dodd, T. R. P. (1992). Responding to symptoms in community pharmacy – urinary tract infections. *Pharmaceutical Journal*, 249, R19.

Bury, M. and Holmes, A. (1990). Quality of life and social support in the very old. *Journal of Ageing Studies*, 4(4), 345–57.

Callahan, C., Huis, N., Ienaber, N., Musach, B. and Tierney, W. (1994). Longitudinal study of depression and health services: use among elderly primary care patients. *Journal of the American Geriatrics Society*, 42(8), 833–8.

Calnan, M. (1983). Social networks and patterns of help-seeking behaviour. *Social Science and Medicine*, 17(2), 25–8.

Calnan, M. (1989). Control over health and patterns of health related behaviour. *Social Science and Medicine*, 29(2), 131–6.

Calnan, M. and Gabe, J. (1991). Recent developments in general practice. In J. Gabe, M. Calnan and M. Bury (eds) *The Sociology of the Health Service*. London: Routledge.

Calnan, S. and Cant, M. (1992). Using private health insurance: a study of lay decisions to seek professional medical help. *Sociology of Health and Illness*, 14(1), 39–56.

Calva, J. (1996). Antibiotic use in a periurban community in Mexico – a household and drugstore survey. *Social Science and Medicine*, 42(8), 1121–8.

Campbell, S. M. and Roland, M. O. (1996). Why do people consult the doctor? *Family Practice*, 13, 75–83.

Cantrill, J. A., Johannesson, B., Nicolson, M. and Noyce, P. R. (1996). Management of minor ailments in primary school children in rural and urban areas. *Child: care, health and development*, 22 (3), 167–74.

Capewell, S. (1996). The continuing rise in emergency admissions. *British Medical Journal*, 312, 991–2.

Cartwright, A. (1979). Minor illness in the surgery: a response to a trivial, ill-defined or inappropriate service? In *Management of Minor Illness*. London: King's Fund.

Cartwright, A. and Smith, C. (1988). *Elderly People, their Medicines, and their Doctors*. London: Routledge.

Castro, R. (1995). The subjective experience of health and illness in Ocuituco: a case study. *Social Science and Medicine*, 3(1), 189–93.

Chapple, A. (1995). Hysterectomy. British NHS services and private patients have very different experiences. *Journal of Advanced Nursing*, 22(5), 900–6.

Cherkin, D., Grothaus, L. and Wagner, E. H. (1992). Is magnitude of co-payment effect related to income? *Social Science and Medicine*, 34(1), 33–41.

Cherkin, D., Deyo, R., Street, J., Hunt, M. and Barlow, W. (1996) Pitfalls of patient education – Limited success of a program for back pain in primary care. *Spine*, 21(3), 345–55.

Clausen, J. and Yarrow, M. (1955). Paths to the mental hospital. *Journal of Social Issues*, 11, 25–33.

Cleary, P. (1989). The demand and need for mental health services. In C. A. Taube, D. Mechanic and A. Hohmann (eds) *The Future of Mental Health Services Research*. Washington, DC: Institute of Mental Health.

Consumers' Association (1994). Vital checks are still not being made. *Which? Way to Health*.

Cook, D. G., Morris, J. K., Walker, M. and Shaper, A. G. (1990). Consultation rates among middle aged men in general practice over three years. *British Medical Journal*, 301, 647–50.

Cooper, L. (1997). Myalgicencephalomyelitis and the medical encounter. *Sociology of Health and Illness*, 19(2), 186–208.

Cornford, C. S., Moran, M. and Ridsdale, L. (1993). Why do mothers consult when their children cough? *Family Practice*. 10(2), 193–6.

Cornwell, J. (1984). *Hard Earned Lives: Accounts of Health and Illness from East London*. London: Tavistock.

Coulter, A. (1997). Partnerships with patients: the pros and cons of shared clinical decision making. *Journal of Health Services Research and Policy*, 2, 112–21.

Courtenay, M. J., Curwen, M. P., Dawe, D., Robinson, J. and Stern, M. J. (1974). Frequent attendance in a family practice, *Journal of Royal College of General Practitioners*, 24, 251–61.

Cowie, W. (1976). The cardiac patient's perception of his heart attack. *Social Science and Medicine*, 10, 87–96.

CSR5 (1997). Shortening patient pathways to care through better use of communication technology Sub group on Direct services in the NHS. (Unpublished report.)

Culyer, A. J. (1995). Need: The idea won't do – but we still need it. *Social Science and Medicine*, 40(6), 727–30.

Cunningham-Burley, S. (1990). Mothers' beliefs about the perceptions of their children's illness. In S. Cunningham-Burley and N. McKeggency (eds) *Readings in Medical Sociology*, 85–109.

Cunningham-Burley, S. and Irvine, S. (1987). 'And have you done anything so far ?' An examination of lay treatment of children's symptoms. *British Medical Journal*, 295, 700–2.

Cunningham-Burley, S. and Maclean, U. (1987). The role of the chemist in primary health care for children with minor complaints. *Social Science and Medicine*, 24, 371–7.

D'Arcy, P. F., Irwin, D. G. and Clarke, D. (1980). Role of the general practice pharmacist in primary health care. *Pharmaceutical Journal*, 224, 539–42.

Davison, C., Davey-Smith, G. and Frankel, S. (1991). Lay epidemiology and the prevention paradox: the implications of coronary candidacy for health education. *Sociology of Health and Illness*, 13(1), 1–19.

De Swaan, A. (1990). *The Management of Normality*. London: Routledge.

Dean, K. (1986). Lay care in illness. *Social Science and Medicine*, 22(2), 275–84.

Dean, K. (1989). Self-care components of lifestyles: the importance of gender attitudes and the social situation. *Social Science and Medicine*, 29(2), 137–52.

Dean, K., Holst, E. and Wagner, M. (1983). Self-care of common illnesses in Denmark. *Medical Care*, 21, 1012.

Del Mar, A. R. (letter) (1996). Recorded consultations for children under five have increased considerably in general practice. *British Medical Journal*, 313, 1334.

Dennis, K. (1990). Patients control and the information imperative. *Nursing Research*, 39(3), 162–6.

Department of Health (1988). *The Health of the Nation*. London: HMSO.

Department of Health (1996). *Choice and Opportunity. Primary Care: The Future*. London: DoH.

Department of Health (1997). *The New NHS: Modern Dependable*. London: HMSO.

Department of Health (1998). *Our Healthier Nation*. London: HMSO.

Dingwall, R. (1971). *Aspects of Illness*. London: Martin Robertson.

Dowrick, C. (1992). Why do the O'Sheas consult so often? An exploration of complex family illness behaviour. *Social Science and Medicine*, 34(5), 491–7.

Dowrick, C., May, R., Richardson, M. and Bundred, P. (1996). The biopsychosocial model of general practice: rhetoric or reality? *British Journal of General Practice*, 46, 105–7.

Doyal, L. and Gough, I. (1991). *A Theory of Social Needs: Review of Philosophical Literature on Needs*. London: Macmillan.

Duffy, M. (1993). Social networks and social support of recently divorced women. *Journal of Public Health Nursing*, 10(1), 19–24.

Dukes, G. and Helsing, E. (1992). Food and drugs: the perils of plenty. *World Health*, 13, 218–21.

Dunnell, K. and Cartwright, A. (1972). *Medicine Takers, Prescribers and Hoarders*. London: Routledge and Kegan Paul.

Editorial (1994). Over the counter drugs. *Lancet*, 343, 1374–5.

Egan, K. J. and Beaton, R. (1987). Response to symptoms in healthy, low utilizers of the health care system. *Journal of Psychosometric Research*, 31, 11–21.

Electoral Reform Ballot Services (1992). *Your Services for the Future: Survey of GP Opinion, UK report.*

Eliot, T. S. (1934). Burnt Norton.

Elsenhans, V., Marquardt, C. and Bledsore, T. (1995). Use of self care manual shifts utilization pattern. *Health Maintenance Practice*, 9(2), 87–90.

Elliot-Binns, C. (1973). An analysis of lay medicine. *Journal of Royal College of General Practitioners*, 23, 255.

Elliott-Binns, C. P. (1986). An analysis of lay medicine: fifteen years later. *Journal of the Royal College of General Practitioners*, 36, 291–4.

Ellis, R. P. and McGuire, T. G. (1986). Cost-sharing and patterns of mental health care utilization. *Journal of Human Resources*, 21(3), 359–79.

Entwistle, V., Sheldon, T., Sowden, A. and Watt, I. (forthcoming). Evidence informed patient choice: practical issues of involving patients in decisions about health care technologies. *International Journal of Technology Assessment in Health Care.*

Eraker, S. A., Kirscht, J. P. and Becker, M. H. (1984). Understanding and improving patient compliance. *Annals of Internal Medicine*, 100(2), 258–68.

Erwin, J., Britten, N. and Jones, R. (1997). General practitioners' views on the OTC availability of H2 antagonists. *British Journal of General Practice*, 47, 99–102.

Estroff, S. E. and Zimmer, Z. (1994). The influence of social networks and social support on violence with persons with serious mental illness. *Hospital and Community Psychiatry*, 45(7), 669–79.

Evans, R. G. (1990). 'The doc in the night-time': medical practice variations and health policy. In T. F. Andersen and G. Mooney (eds) *The Challenge of Medical Practice Variations.* Basingstoke: Macmillan.

Evans, S. W. and John, D. N. (1997). Who would the public ask for advice on selected symptoms? *Pharmaceutical Journal*, 260, 16.

Evans, S. W., John, D. N. and Bloor, M. (1996). Patterns and compliance with referrals made by community pharmacists in response to clients presenting with symptoms. *Pharmaceutical Journal*, 257, R15.

Evans, S. W., John, D. N., Bloor, M. and Luscombe, D. K. (1995). Utilisation of the advice offered by community pharmacists to clients presenting with symptoms. *Pharmaceutical Journal*, 255, R29.

Evans, S. W., John, D. N., Bloor, M. J. and Luscombe, D. K. (1997). Use of non-prescription advice offered to the public by community pharmacists. *International Journal of Pharmacy Practice*, 5, 16–25.

Eyles, J. and Donovan, J. (1990). *The Social Effects of Health Policy.* Aldershot: Avebury.

Feenberg, A. L., Licht, J. M., Kane, K. P., Moran, K., Smith, R. A. (1996). The online patient meeting. *Journal of Neurological Sciences*, 139 (Supplement), 129–31.

Ferkenhoff, E. (1995). *Patient Heal Thyself.* Special Report, 16 October. Chicago: Crain Communications.

Field, D. (1976). The social definition of illness. In D. Tuckett (ed.) *An Introduction to Medical Sociology*. London: Tavistock.

Finlayson, A. (1976). Social networks as coping resources, lay help and consultation patterns used by women in husbands' post infarction career. *Social Science and Medicine*, 10, 97–103.

Finney, J. W., Riley, A. W. and Cataldo, M. (1991). Psychology in primary health care. *Journal of Paediatric Psychology*, 16(4), 447–61.

Fisher, C. M., Corrigan, O. I. and Henman, M. C. (1991). A study of community pharmacy practice: non-prescribed medicine sales and counselling. *Journal of Social and Administrative Pharmacy*, 8, 69–75.

Fitzgibbon, J., Murphy, D., O'Shea, T. and Kelleher, C. (1997). Chronic debilitating fatigue in Irish general practice: a survey of general practitioners' experience. *British Journal of General Practice*, 47(423), 618–23.

Fitzpatrick, R., Hinton, J., Newman, S., Scambler, G. and Thompson, J. (eds) (1986). *The Experience of Illness*. London: Tavistock.

Foot, M. (1975). *Aneurin Bevan, 1945–60*. London: Paladin.

Freer, C. (1980). Self-care: a health diary study. *Medical Care*, 18, 853–61.

Freidson, E. (1960). Client control and medical practice. *American Journal of Sociology*, 65, 374–82.

Freidson, E. (1970). *Profession of Medicine: A Study in the Sociology of Applied Knowledge*. New York: Dodd Mead.

Frewer, L., Sheperd, R. and Sparks, P. (1994). The interrelationship between perceived knowledge, control and risk associated with a range of food hazards. *Journal of Food Safety*, 14(1), 19–40.

Fulder, S. J. and Munro, R. (1985). Complementary medicine in the United Kingdom – patients, practitioners and consultations. *Lancet*, 2(8454), 542–5.

Furnham, A. (1994). Explaining health and illness: lay perceptions on current and future health, the causes of illness, and the nature of recovery. *Social Science and Medicine*, 39(5), 715–25.

Furnham, A. and Forey, J. (1994). The attitudes, behaviours and beliefs of patients of conventional vs complementary medicine. *Journal of Clinical Psychology*, 50(3), 458–569.

Gabe, J., Gustafsson, U. and Bury, M. (1991). Mediating illness – newspaper coverage of tranquilizer dependence. *Sociology of Health and Illness*, 13(3), 332–53.

Gallagher, M., Huddart, T. and Henderson, B. (1998). Telephone triage of acute illness by a practice nurse in general practice: outcomes of care. *British Journal of General Practice*, 48, 1141–5.

Gerrard, T. J. and Riddell, J. D. (1988). Difficult patients: black holes and secrets. *British Medical Journal*, 297, 530–2.

Ghalamkari, H. H., Rees, J. E. and Saltrese-Taylor, A. (1995). Clients' response to health promotion advice given by community pharmacists. *Pharmaceutical Journal*, 255, R19.

Giachello, A., Fleming, G. and Andersen, R. (1982). *Self-care Practices in the United States*, Research Project Report. Chicago: Centre for Health Administration Studies, University of Chicago.

Gibson, P., Henry, R., Vimpani, G. and Halliday, J. *et al.* (1995). Asthma knowledge, attitudes and quality of life in adolescents. *Archives of Disease in Childhood*, 73(4), 321–6.

Giddens, A. (1991). *Modernity and Self-Identity: Self and Society in the Late Modern Age*. Cambridge: Polity.

Gillam, S. (1990). Ethnicity and the use of health services. *Postgraduate Medical Journal*, 66, 989–93.

Goffman, E. (1961). *Asylums*. Harmondsworth: Penguin.

Goodburn, E., Mattossinho, S., Mongi, P. and Waterson, T. (1991). Management of childhood diarrhoea by pharmacists and parents: is Britain lagging behind the Third World? *British Medical Journal*, 302, 440–3.

Gourash, N. (1978). Help-seeking: a review of the literature. *American Journal of Community Psychology*, 6(5), 413–23.

Graham, H. (1987). Women's smoking and family health. *Social Science and Medicine*, 25(1), 47–56.

Green, J. and Dale, J. (1992). Primary care in accident and emergency and general practice: a comparison. *Social Science and Medicine*, 35(8), 987–1005.

Greimel, E., Padilla, G. and Grant, M. (1997). *Acta Oncology*, 36(2), 141–50.

Gribben, B. (1992). Do access factors affect utilisation of general practitioner services in South Auckland. *New Zealand Medical Journal*, 105, 453–5.

Hallam, L. (1994). Primary health care outside normal working hours: review of published work. *British Medical Journal*, 308, 249–53.

Hallam, L. and Cragg, D. (1994). Organisation of primary care services outside normal working hours. *British Medical Journal*, 309(6969), 1621–3.

Hallam, L. and Henthorne, K. (1998). *Co-operatives and their Primary Care Emergency Centres: Organisation and Impact*. Manchester: National Primary Care Research and Development Centre.

Ham, C. (1992). *Health Policy in Britain: The Politics and Organisation of the National Health Service*. Basingstoke: Macmillan.

Ham, C. (1998). Financing the NHS. *British Medical Journal*, 316, 237–38.

Hannay, D. (1979). *The Symptom Iceberg. A Study of Community Health*. London: Routledge and Kegan Paul.

Hardisty, B. (1982). Do assistants take the pharmacists' role in counter prescribing? *Chemist and Druggist*, 218, 804–8.

Hargie, O., Morrow, N. and Woodman, C. (1992). Consumer perceptions of attitudes to community pharmacy services. *Pharmaceutical Journal*, 249, 688–91.

Hassell, K., Harris, J., Rogers, J., Noyce, P. R. and Wilkinson, J. (1996). *The Role and Contribution of Pharmacy in Primary Care*. Manchester: National Primary Care Research and Development Centre.

Hassell, K., Noyce, P. R., Rogers, A., Harris, J. and Wilkinson, J. (1997). A pathway to the GP: the pharmaceutical 'consultation' as a first port of call in primary health care. *Family Practice*, 14 (6), 458–61.

Hassell, K., Noyce, P. R., Rogers, A., Harris, J. and Wilkinson, J. (forthcoming). Demand for advice across the chemist's counter: the nature of the 'pharmaceutical consultation'. *Journal of Health Services Research and Policy*.

Haug, M. and Lavin, B. (1983). Utilization mode: a review. Paper presented at the American Sociological Association Meeting.

Hayes, A. and Livingstone, C. R. (1990). Advice on prescribed medicines in community pharmacies. *Pharmaceutical Journal*, 244, 239–41.

Hertzlich, C. and Piernet, J. (1987). *Illness and Self in Society*. Baltimore: Johns Hopkins University Press.

Hibbert, D. and Elliott, J. (1996). *An Assessment of Need for Community Pharmaceutical Services in Dorset*. Manchester: Pharmacy Practice Research and Resource Centre.

Higgins, J. and Ruddell, S. (1991). Working for a better alternative. *Health Service Journal*, 24 July, 26–8.

Hirschfield, A., Wolfson, D. J. and Swetman, S. (1994). Location of community pharmacies: a rational approach to using geographic information systems. *International Journal of Pharmacy Practice*, 3, 42–52.

Holloway, S. W. F. (1991). *Royal Pharmaceutical Society of Great Britain 1841–1991. A Political and Social History*. London: Pharmaceutical Press.

Hoog, S. (1992). The self-medication market – a literature review. *Journal of Social and Administrative Pharmacy*, 9, 123–37.

Hopton, J. and Dlugolecka, M. (1995). Need and demand for primary health care: a comparative survey approach. *British Medical Journal*, 310, 1369–73.

Horner, B., Scheibe, K. and Stine, S. (1996). Cocaine abuse and attention–deficit hyperactivity disorder implications of adult symptomatology. *Psychology of Addictive Behaviours*, 10(1), 55–60.

Howlett, B., Waqar, I.-U. Ahmad and Murray, R. (1991). An examination of white, Asian and Afro-Caribbean people's concepts of health and illness causation. Paper presented at the annual conference of the *British Sociological Association*, Manchester, 25–28 March.

Hughes, I. (1997). Can you keep from crying by considering things? Some arguments against cognitive therapy for depression. *Clinical Psychology Forum*, 104 , 23–8.

Huygen, F., van der Hoogen, H. and Neefs, W. (1983). Gezondheid en ziekte, een onderzoek van gezinnen Ned. Tijdschr. *Geneeskunde*, 127, 1612.

Ignatieff, M. (1994). *The Needs of Strangers*. London: Vintage.

Illich, I. (1976). *Limits to Medicine: Medical Nemesis: The Exploration of Health*. London: Marion Boyars.

Ingham, J. and Miller, P. (1982). Consulting with mild symptoms in general practice. *Social and Psychiatric Epidemiology*, 17, 77–88.

Irvine, S. and Cunningham-Burley, S. (1991). Mothers' concepts of normality, behavioural change and illness in their children. *British Journal of General Practice*, 41(350), 371–4.

Jarman, F. (1995). Communication problems: a patient's view. *Nursing Times*, 91(18), 30–1.

Jepson, M. H. and Strickland-Hodge, B. (1993). Patient's choice of pharmacy, the importance of PMRs and patient registration. *Pharmaceutical Journal*, 251, R35.

Jepson, M., Jesson, J., Kendall, H. and Pocock, R. (1991). *Consumer Expectations of Community Pharmaceutical Services: A Research Report for the Department of Health.* Birmingham: Pharmacy Practice Group and Social and Consumer Research Unit, Aston University, MEL Research, Aston Science Park.

Jesson, J., Jepson, M., Pocock, R., Sadler, S. and Dunbar, P. (1994). *Ethnic Minority Consumers of Community Pharmaceutical Services: A Report for the Department of Health.* Birmingham: Pharmacy Practice Research Group, Aston University and MEL Research, Aston Science Park.

John, D. N., Evans, S. W. and Hammersley, C. M. (1995). Investigation of the opinions of prescription customers on new non-prescription medicines. *Proceedings of the UK Clinical Pharmacy Association*, 50–1.

Kadushin, C. (1966). The friends and supporters of psychotherapy: on social circles in urban life. *American Sociological Review*, 31, 786–802.

Kahneman, D. and Tversky, A. (1979). Prospect theory: an analysis of decision under risk. *Econometria*, 49, 263–91.

Kahneman, D. and Tversky, A. (1984). Choices, values and frames. *American Psychologist*, 39, 341–50.

Karlsson, H., Letitinen, V. and Jonkamaa, M. (1995). Are frequent attenders of primary health care distressed? *Scandinavian Journal of Primary Health Care*, 13(1), 32–8.

Karpf, A. (1988). *Doctoring the Media.* London: Routledge.

Kasl, S. and Cobb, S. (1996). Health behaviour, illness behaviour and sick role behaviour. *Archives of Environmental Research*, 12(2), 246–7.

Kayne, S. and Reeves, A. (1994). Sports care and the pharmacists – an opportunity not to be missed. *Pharmaceutical Journal*, 253, 66–7.

Kendrick, S. (1996). The pattern of increase in emergency hospital admissions in Scotland. *Health Bulletin*, 54, 101–9.

Kiely, B. G. and McPherson, I. (1986). Stress, self-help packages in primary care: a controlled trial evaluation. *Journal of the Royal College of General Practitioners*, 36, 307–9.

Klein, R. (1995). *The New Politics of the NHS.* London: Longman.

Klein, R., Day, P., Redmayne, S. (1996). *Managing Scarcity: Priority Setting and Rationing in the NHS.* Buckingham: Open University Press.

Klemm, P., Reppert, K., and Visich, L. (1998) A non-traditional cancer support group. *The Internet Computers in Nursing*, 16(1), 31–6.

Knapp, D. A. and Knapp, D. E. (1972). Decision-making and self medication: preliminary findings. *American Journal of Hospital Pharmacy*, 29, 1004–12.

Komter, A. E. (1996). Reciprocity as a principle of exclusion. *Sociology*, 30(2), 299–316.

Konning, C., Maille, A., Stevens, I. and Dekker, F. (1995). Patients' opinions on respiratory care: do doctors fulful their needs. *Journal of Asthma*, 32(5), 355–63.

Kookier, S. (1995). Exploring the iceberg of morbidity: a comparison of different survey methods for assessing the occurrence of everyday illness. *Social Science Medicine*, 41(3), 317–32.

Kroeger, A. (1983). Anthropological and sociomedical health care research in developing countries. *Social Science and Medicine*, 17(3), 147–61.

Kronefield, J. (1979). Self care as a panacea for the ills of the health care system: an assessment. *Social Science and Medicine*, 13a, 269.

Krska, J. and Kennedy, E. (1996). Expectations and experiences of customers purchasing OTC medicines in pharmacies in the north of Scotland. *Pharmaceutical Journal*, 256, 354–6.

Krska, J., Greenwood, R. and Howitt, E. P. (1994). Audit of advice provided in response to symptoms. *Pharmaceutical Journal*, 252, 93–6.

Lattymer, V., Glasper, H. and George, S. (1995). The views of general practitioners on the provision of out of hours primary medical care. *Health and Social Care in the Community*, 3(1), 58–61.

Leavy, R. (1983). Social support and psychological disorder – a review. *Journal of Community Psychology*, 11, 13–21.

Leibowitz, A. (1989). Substitution between prescribed and OTC medications. *Medical Care*, 27, 85–94.

Lerman, C., Schwartz, M., Miller, S. and Daly, M. (1996). A randomized trial of breast cancer risk counselling. *Health Psychology*, 15(2), 75–83.

Leventhal, H. and Nerenz, D. (1985). The assessment of illness cognition. In P. Karoly (ed.) *Measurement Strategies in Health Psychology*. New York: Wiley.

Levin, L. S. (1976). The layperson as the primary health care practitioner. *Public Health Reports*, 91, 206.

Levitt, R. and Wall, A. (1991). *The Reorganised National Health Service*, 4th edition. London: Longman.

Light, D. W. (1997). From managed competition to managed cooperation: theory and lessons from the British Experience. *Milbank Quarterly*, 75(3), 297.

Light, D. (1998). Is NHS purchasing serious? An American perspective. *British Medical Journal*, 316, 217–21.

Little, P., Williamson, G., Warner, G., Gould, C., Gantley, M. and Kinmouth, A. L. (1997). Open randomised trial of prescribing strategies in managing sore throat. *British Medical Journal*, 3(314), 8 March.

Living in Great Britain: The 1995 General Household Survey. London: HMSO.

Livingstone, C. (1995). The views of elderly people on information from community pharmacists about prescribed medicines. *Pharmaceutical Journal*, 255, R7.

Livingstone, C., Williamson, V. and Winn, S. (1993). Will customers accept community pharmacy's extended role? *Institute of Pharmacy Management*, 15(2), 262–6.

LoGerfo, J., Moore, S. and Thomas, S. (1981) Letter. *Journal of the American Medical Association*, 2245(4), 342.

Lomas, J. (1997). Reluctant rationers: public input to health care priorities. *Journal of Health Services Research and Policy*, 2(2), 103–21.

Ludwick, R. (1992). Registered nurses' knowledge and practices of teaching and performing breast exams among elderly women. *Cancer Nursing*, 15(1), 61–7.

Lynch, M. (1994). Preparing children for day surgery. *Children's Health Care*, 23(2), 75–85.

Lyons, R., Perry, I., Perry, M. and Littlepage, B. (1994). Evidence for the validity of the short-form 36 questionnaire in an elderly population. *Age and Ageing*, 23(3), 182–4.

McCormick, A., Fleming, D. and Charlton, J. (1995). *Morbidity Statistics from General Practice: Fourth National Study 1991–1992*. London: HMSO.

Macdonald, E. and Macdonald, J. (1992). How do local doctors react to a hospice? *Health Bulletin*, 50(5), 351–5.

McElnay, J. C. and Dickson, F. C. (1994). Purchase from community pharmacies of OTC medicines by elderly patients. *Pharmaceutical Journal*, 253, R15.

McElnay, J. C., Nicholl, A. J. and Grainger-Rousseau, T. J. (1993). The role of the community pharmacist – a survey of public opinion in Northern Ireland. *International Journal of Pharmacy Practice*, 2, 95–100.

Mackay, H. (1990). Patients who consult a doctor infrequently. *Update*, 41, 11–12, 30.

Mackillop, W., Palmer, M., O'Sullivan, B., Ward, G., Steele, R. and Dotsikas, G. (1989). Clinical trials in cancer: the role of surrogate patients in defining what constitutes an acceptable clinical experiment. *British Journal of Cancer*, 59(3), 388–95.

McKinlay, J. (1972). Some approaches and problems in the study of the use of services – an overview. *Journal of Health and Social Behaviour*, 13(15), 29–46.

McKinlay, J. (1973). Social networks, lay consultation and help seeking behaviour. *Social Forces*, 51, 275–92.

McLean, J. and Peitroni, P. (1990). Self care – who does best? *Social Science and Medicine*, 30(5), 591–6.

Magi, M. and Allander, E. (1981). Towards a theory of perceived and medically defined need. *Sociology of Health and Illness*, 3(1), 25–33.

Malone, R. (1995). Heavy users of emergency services: social construction of a policy problem. *Social Science and Medicine*, 40(4), 469–77.

Mark, A. and Elliott, R. (forthcoming). De-marketing dysfunctional demand in health developing practices in the UK National Health Service. *International Journal of Health Planning and Management.*

Marteau, T. (1989). Framing of information: its influence upon decisions of doctors and patients. *British Journal of Social Psychology*, 28, 89–94.

May, C. (1997). Degrees of freedom: reflexivity, self-identity and self-help. *Self, Agency and Society*, 1(1), 42–54.

May, C. and Mead, N. (in press). Patient-centredness: a history. In C. Dowrich and L. Frith (eds). *Ethical Problems in General Practice.* London: Routledge.

Meade, C., McKinney, W. and Barnas, G. (1994). Educating patients with limited literacy skills: the effectiveness of printed and videotaped material about colon cancer. *American Journal of Public Health*, 84(1), 119–21.

Mechanic, D. (1961). The concept of illness behaviour. *Journal of Chronic Diseases*, 15, 189.

Mechanic, D. (1979). Correlates of physician utilization: why do major multivariate studies of physician utilization find trivial psychosocial and organizational effects? *Journal of Health and Social Behaviour*, 20, 387.

Mechanic, D. (1980). The experience and reporting of common physical complaints. *Journal of Health and Social Behaviour*, 21, 146.

Mechanic, D. (1990). The role of sociology in health affairs. *Health Affairs*, 9(1), 85–97.

Mechanic, D. (1995). Sociological dimensions of illness behaviour. *Social Science and Medicine*, 41(9), 1207–16.

Medalie, J., Stange, K., Zyzanski, S. and Goldbourt, U. (1992). The importance of bio-psychosocial factors in the development of duodenal ulcers in a cohort of middle-aged men. *American Journal of Epidemiology*, 136(10), 1280–7.

Meininger, J. C. (1986). Sex differences in factors associated with the use of medical care and alternative illness behaviours. *Social Science and Medicine*, 22(3), 285–92.

Meredith, P. (1993). Patient participation in decision-making and consent to treatment in the case of general surgery. *Sociology of Health and Illness*, 15(3), 315–36.

Mesters, I., Meerlens, R. and Mosterol, N. (1991). Multi-disciplinary co-operation in primary care for asthmatic children. *Social Science and Medicine*, 32(1), 657–70.

Milburn, L. J., Dunbar, P. E. and Kendall, H. E. (1990). Factors influencing pharmacy patronage in the West Midlands. *Pharmaceutical Journal*, 245, R19.

Miles, A. (1991). *Women, Health and Medicine.* Buckingham: Open University Press.

Miller, C. and Hart, G. (1995). Reduced disease prevalence at a sexually transmitted diseases clinic during a mass media campaign. *Venereology International Journal of Sexual Health*, 49, 59–64.

Mitra, J., Saha, J. and Chaudhuri, R. (1993). Drug consumption pattern in low socio-economic groups in an urban community. *Indian Journal of Public Health* (India), 37(1), 16–22.

Monroe, S., Simons, A. and Thase, M. (1991). Onset of depression and time of treatment entry – roles of life stress. *Journal of Consulting and Clinical Psychology*, 59(4), 566–73.

Moon, G. (1995). (RE) placing research on health and health care. *Health and Place*, 2(1), 1–4.

Moore, S., LoGerfo, J. and Inui, T. (1980). Effect of a self-care book on physician visits: a randomized trial. *Journal of the American Medical Association*, 243(22), 2317–20.

Morgan, M. (1988). Managing hypertension – beliefs and responses to medication among cultural groups. *Sociology of Health and Illness*, 10(4), 561–78.

Morrell, D., Gage, H. and Robinson, N. (1971). Symptoms in general practice. *Journal of the Royal College of General Practitioners*, 21, 32–43.

Morrissey, J. (1997). Managed care: on call modern health care. *Modern Health Care*, 25 August, 50–3.

Morrissey, J. (1997). On Call Foundation health system's sophisticated telephone triage centre gains popularity with patients and physicians. *Modern Health Care*, 25 August, 25–8.

Morrow, N., Hargie, O. and Woodman, C. (1993). Consumer perceptions of and attitudes to the advice-giving role of community pharmacists. *Pharmaceutical Journal*, 251, 25–7.

Morse, E., Simon, P., Baus, S., Balson, P. and Osofsky, H. (1992). Cofactors of substance use among male street prostitutes. *Journal of Drug Issues*, 22(4), 977–94.

Mottram, D. R., Ford, J. L., Markey, B. and Mitchelson, K. (1989). Public perceptions of community pharmacy. *Pharmaceutical Journal*, 253, R14–17.

Mueller, D. (1980). Social networks: a promising direction for research on the relationship of the social environment to psychiatric disorder. *Social Science and Medicine*, 14a(3), 147–61.

Muellen, K. (1992). A question of balance: health behaviour and work context among male Glaswegians. *Sociology of Health and Illness*, 14, 173–98.

Mukerjee, D. and Blane, D. B. (1990). Pharmaceutical service delivery by community pharmacies in areas of contrasting medical provision. *Social Science and Medicine*, 31, 1277–80.

Mulleady, G. and Green, J. (1985). Syringe sharing among London drug abusers. *Lancet* II, 1425.

Murray, J. and Sheperd, S. (1993). Alternative or additional medicine – an exploratory study in general practice. *Social Science and Medicine*, 37(8), 983–8.

Murray, J. and Williams, P. (1986). Self-reported illness and general practice consultations in Asian born and British born residents of West London. *Social Psychiatry and Psychiatric Epidemiology*, 21, 139–45.

NAHAT (National Association of Health Authorities and Trusts) (1994). *Emergency Admissions: Managing the Rising Trend*, Briefing No. 74. Birmingham: NAHAT.

National Audit Office (1992). *Community Pharmacies in England: Report by the Comptroller Auditor General*. London: HMSO.

Neal, R. D., Heywood, P. L., Morley, S., Clayden, A. D. and Dowell, A. C. (1998). Frequency of patients' consulting in general practice and workload generated by frequent attenders: comparisons between practices. *British Journal of General Practice*, 48(426), 895–8.

NHS Executive (1996). *Promoting Clinical Effectiveness: A Framework for Action through the NHS*. London: Department of Health.

Nuffield Foundation (1986). *Pharmacy: The Report of the Committee of Inquiry Appointed by the Nuffield Foundation*. London: Nuffield.

O'Dowd, T. C. (1988). Five years of heartsink patients in general practice. *British Medical Journal*, 297, 528–30.

O'Dowd, T., Parker, S. and Kelly, A. (1996). Women's experiences of general practitioners' management of their vaginal symptoms. *British Journal of General Practice*, 46, 415–18.

Oakley, A. (1992). *Motherhood and Social Support*. Oxford: Blackwell.

Oakley, A. (1994). Who cares for health? Social relations, gender and the public health. *Journal of Epidemiology and Community Health*, 48, 427–34.

Offe, C. (1984). *Contradictions of the Welfare State*. London: Hutchinson.

Olin Lauritzen, S. (1997). Notions of child health: mothers' accounts of health in their young babies. *Sociology of Health and Illness*, 19(4), 436–57.

Oliver, M. (1990). *The Politics of Disability*. Basingstoke: Macmillan.

OPCS (1995a). *General Household Survey*. No. 24. London: HMSO.

OPCS (1995b). *Morbidity Statistics from General Practice: Fourth National Study 1991–1992*. London: HMSO.

Øvretveit, J. (1997). Managing the gap between demand and publicly affordable health care in an ethical way. *European Journal of Public Health*, 7(2), 128–35.

Paraskevaidis, E., Kitchener, H. C. and Walker, L. G. (1993). Doctor–patient communication and subsequent mental health in women with gynaecological cancer. *Psycho-oncology*, 2(3), 195–200.

Parsons, T. (1950). Illness and the role of the physician. *American Journal of Orthopsychiatry*, 21, 452–60.

Parsons, T. (1951). *The Social System*. Glencoe, IL: Free Press.

Payne, K., Ryan-Woolley, B. W. and Noyce, P. R. (1996). *The Impact of Deregulation: A Study of Decision-making and Willingness to Pay*. Manchester: Academic Pharmacy Practice Group, University of Manchester.

Pearse, I. and Crocker, L. (1943). *The Peckham Experiment: a Study in the Living Structure of Society*. London: Northamptonshire Printing and Publishing Co.

Pearson, M., Dawson, C., Moore, H. and Spece, S. (1993). Health on borrowed time? Prioritizing and meeting needs in low income households. *Health and Social Care in the Community*, 1, 11–68.

Pedersen, L. and Leese, B. (1997). What will a primary care led NHS mean for GP workload? The problem of the lack of an evidence base in education and debate. *British Medical Journal*, 314(14), 1337–41.

Pencheon, D. (1996). *On Demand*. Working Paper. Cambridge: Institute of Public Health.

Pencheon, D. (1998). Managing demand: Matching demand and supply fairly and efficiently. *British Medical Journal*, 316(7145), 1665–7.

Pescosolido, B. A. (1991). Illness, careers and network ties: a conceptual model of utilization and compliance. *Advances in Medical Sociology*, 2, 161–84.

Pescosolido, B. (1992). Beyond rational choice: the social dynamics of how people seek help. *American Journal of Sociology*, 97(4), 1096–138.

Pescosolido, B. and Boyer, C. (1996). From the community into the treatment system – how people use health services. In A. Horwitz and T. Scheid (eds) *The Sociology of Mental Illness*. New York: Oxford University Press.

Pescosolido, B. A. and Kronenfeld, J. (1995). Health, illness and healing in an uncertain era: challenges on, from and for medical sociology. *Journal of Health and Social Behaviour*, extra issue, 5–33.

Pescosolido, B., Gardner, B. and Lubell, K. (1998). How people get into mental health services: stories of choice, coercion and 'muddling through' from 'first timers'. *Social Science and Medicine*, 46(2), 275–86.

Phillips, K. and Morrison, K., Anderson, R, and Aday, L. (1998). Understanding the context of health care utilization: assessing environmental and provider-related variables in the behavioural model of utilization. *Health Services Research*, 33(3), 571–96.

Pietroni, P. and Chase, H. (1993). Partners of partisans – patient participation at Marylebone Health Centre. *British Journal of General Practice*, 43, 341–4.

Pilgrim, D., Todhunter, C. and Pearson, M. (1997). Accounting for disability: customer feedback or citizen complaints. *Disability and Society*, 12(1), 3–15.

Pill, R. (1987). Models and management: the case of cystitis in women. *Sociology of Health and Illness*, 9(3), 265–86.

Pill, R. and Stott, N. (1985). Preventive procedures and practices among working class women: new data and fresh insights. *Social Science and Medicine*, 21(9), 975–83.

Pini, S., Piccinelli, M. and Zimmermann-Tansella, C. (1995). Social problems as factors affecting medical consultation: a comparison between general practice attenders and community probands with emotional distress. *Psychological Medicine*, 25(1), 33–41.

Plamping, D. and Delamothe, T. (1991). The Citizens' Charter and the NHS. *British Medical Journal*, 303(6796), 203–4.

Pope, C. (1991). Trouble in store: some thoughts on the management of waiting lists. *Sociology of Health and Illness*, 13(2), 194–211.

Povey, T., Dunbar, P. E. and Kendall, H. E. (1990). Pharmacists' perceptions of the factors important to customer loyalty. *Pharmaceutical Journal*, 245, R18.

Prout, A. (1988). Off school sick – mothers' accounts of school sickness absences. *Sociological Review*, 36(4), 765–89.

Pulse (1998). GP World View 'Same-day appointments reduce US consultations', p. 7.

Punamaki, Raija-Leena and Kokko, Simo J. (1995a). Content and predictors of consultation experiences among Finnish primary care patients. *Social Science and Medicine*, 40(2), 231–43.

Punamaki, Raija-Leena and Kokko, Simo J. (1995b). Reasons for consultation and explanations of illness among Finnish primary-care led patients. *Sociology of Health and Illness*, 17(1), 42–64.

Radley, A. (1994). *Making Sense of Illness: The Social Psychology of Health and Disease*. London: Sage.

Rasmussen, C. (1989). Mothers' benefit of a self-care booklet and a self-care educational session at child health centres. *Social Science and Medicine*, 29(2), 205–12.

Reif, L. V., Patton, M. J. and Gold, P. B. (1995). Bereavement, stress and social support in members of a self-help group. *Journal of Community Psychology*, 23(4), 292–306.

Reis, J. and Wrestler, F. (1994). Consumer attitudes towards computer-assisted self-care of the common cold. *Patient Education and Counseling*, 23(1), 55–62.

Rickwood, D. J. and Braithwaite, V. A. (1994). Social-psychological factors affecting help seeking for emotional problems. *Social Science and Medicine*, 39(4), 563–72.

Riessman, C., Whalen, M., Frost, R. and Morgenthau, E. (1991). Romance and help-seeking among college women – it hurts so much to care. *Women and Health*, 17(4), 21–47.

Ritchie, J., Jacoby, A. and Bone, M. (1981). *Access to Primary Health Care. An Enquiry Carried Out on Behalf of the United Kingdom Health Departments*. London: HMSO.

Roberts, H. (1992). Professionals' and parents' perceptions of A-and-E use in a children's hospital. *Sociological Review*, 40(1), 109–31.

Robinson, D. (1971). *The Process of Becoming Ill*. London: Routledge and Kegan Paul.

Robinson, R. and Steiner, A. (1998). *Managed Health Care: US Evidence and Lessons for the NHS*. Buckingham: Open University Press.

Rochaix, L. (1989). Information asymmetry and search in the market for physicians' services. *Journal of Health Economics*, 8(1), 53–84.

Rogers, A. (1990). Policing mental disorder: controversies, myths and realities. *Social Policy and Administration*, 24(3), 226–37.

Rogers, A. and Pilgrim, D. (1995). The risk of resistance: perspectives on the mass childhood immunisation programme. In J. Gabe (ed.) *Medicine, Health and Risk*, Sociology of Health and Illness Monograph. Oxford: Blackwell.

Rogers, A., Pilgrim, D. and Lacey, R. (1993). *Experiencing Psychiatry*. Basingstoke: Macmillan.

Rogers, A., Popay, J., Williams, G. and Latham, M. (1997a). *Health Variations and Health Behaviour: Insights from the Qualitative Literature*, Health Variations Report I. London: Health Education Authority.

Rogers, A., Pilgrim, D. and Latham, M. (1997b). *Understanding and Promoting Mental Health*. London: Health Education Authority.

Rogers, A., Chapple, C. and Halliwell, S. (1998). The influence of paid and unpaid work on helpseeking for primary care. *Social Sciences and Health*, 4(3), 188–99.

Rogers, A., Hassell, K., Noyce, P. R., Harris, J. and Wilkinson, J. (forthcoming). Variations in advice giving in community pharmacy. *Health and Place*.

Roland, M. and Dixon, M. (1989). Randomized controlled trial of an educational booklet for patients' presentations within general practice. *Journal of the Royal College of General Practitioners*, 39, 244–6.

Roland, M. and Wilkin, D. (1996). Rationale for moving towards a primary care led NHS. In *What is the Future for a Primary Care Led NHS*. NPCRDC, Oxford: Radcliffe Medical Press.

Rosenstock, I. (1966). Why people use health services. *Milbank Memorial Fund Quarterly*, 44, 94–127.

Roth, J. A. (1963). *Timetables*. Cleveland: Bobbs-Merill.

Rowlands, O., Singleton, N., Maher, J. and Higgins, V. (1997). *Living in Britain: Results from the 1995 General Household Survey*. London: HMSO.

Royal Pharmaceutical Society of Great Britain (1996). *Community Pharmacy: The Choice Is Yours. Access to and Usage of Community Pharmacies – the Customer's View*. London: RPSGB.

Royal Pharmaceutical Society of Great Britain and Department of Health (1992). *Pharmaceutical Care: The Future for Community Pharmacy. Report of the Joint Working Party on the Future Role of the Community Pharmaceutical Services*. London: RPSGB.

Rudat, K. (1994). *Health and Lifestyles: Black and Minority Ethnic Groups in England*. London: Health Education Authority.

Saks, M. (ed.) (1992). *Alternative Medicine in Britain*. Oxford: Clarendon.

Salloway, J. and Dillon, P. (1973). A comparison of family networks in health care utilization. *Journal of Comparative Family Services*, 4, 131–42.

Saunders, S. (1993). Applicants' experience of the process of seeking therapy. *Psychotherapy*, 30(4), 554–63.

Scambler, A. and Scambler, G. (1984). The illness iceberg and aspects of consulting behaviour. In R. Fitzpatrick *et al.* (eds) *The Experience of Illness*. London: Tavistock.

Scambler, A., Scambler, G. and Craig, D. (1981). Kinship and friendship networks and women's demand for primary care. *Journal of the Royal College of General Practitioners*, 31, 746–50.

Schafheutle, E. I., Cantrill, J. A., Nicholson, M. and Noyce, P. R. (1996). Insights into the choice between self-medication and a doctor's prescription: a study of hay fever sufferers. *International Journal of Pharmacy Practice*, 4, 156–61.

Schommer, J. C. and Wiederhold, J. B. (1992). Pharmacists' perceptions of patients' needs for counselling. *American Journal of Hospital Pharmacy*, 51, 478–85.

Scott, A., King, M. and Shiell, A. (1995a). *Factors Influencing Decision Making in General Practice: The Feasibility of Analysing Secondary Data. Report to the Evaluation Steering Group, General Practice Evaluation Programme*. CHERE Discussion Paper Series. Centre for Health Economics Research and Evaluation.

Scott, S., Deary, I. and Pelosi, S. (1995b). General practitioners' attitudes to patients with a self-diagnosis of myalgicencephalomyelitis. *British Medical Journal*, 310, 508.

Seedhouse, D. (1994). *Fortress NHS: A Philosophical Review of the NHS*. Chichester: Wiley.

Segall, A. (1990). A community survey of self-medication activities. *Medical Care*, 28, 301–10.

Segall, A. and Goldstein, J. (1989). Exploring the correlates of self-provided health care behaviour. *Social Science and Medicine*, 29(2), 153–61.

Selznick, P. (1957). *Leadership in Administration*. London: Harper and Row.

Sharma, U. (1990). Using alternative therapies: marginal medicine and central concerns. In P. Abbott and G. Payne (eds) *New Directions in the Sociology of Health*. London: Falmer Press.

Sheaff, R. (1996). *The Need for Health Care*. London: Routledge.

Shuval, J., Janetz, R. and Shye, D. (1989). Self-care in Israel: physicians' views and perspectives. *Social Science and Medicine*, 29(2), 233–44.

Shye, D., Mullooly, J., Freeborn, K. and Pope, C. (1995). Gender differences in the relationship between social network support and mortality – a longitudinal study of an elderly cohort. *Social Science and Medicine*, 41(7), 935–47.

Singh, A. K., Moldu, K., Trell, E. and Wigertz, O. (1992). Computers, methods and programmes. *Biomedicine*, 37(5), 55–64.

Skelton, J. and Pennebaker, J. (1982). The psychology of physical symptoms and sensations. In G. Sanders and J. Suls (eds) *Social Psychology of Health and Illness*. Hillsdale: Lawrence Erlbaum Associates.

Smaje, C. and Le Grand, J. (1997). Ethnicity, equity and use of health services in the British NHS. *Social Science and Medicine,* 45(3), 485–96.

Smart, B. (1992). *Modern Conditions and Post Modern Controversies*. London: Routledge.

Smith, F. J. (1990a). Factors important to clients when seeking the advice of a pharmacist. *Pharmaceutical Journal*, 244, 692–3.

Smith, F. J. (1990b). Presentation of clinical symptoms to community pharmacists in London. *Journal of Social and Administrative Pharmacy*, 7, 221–4.

Smith, F. J. (1992). A study of the advisory and health promotion activity of community pharmacists. *Health Education Journal*, 51, 68–71.

Smith, F. J. (1993). Referral of clients by community pharmacists in primary care consultations. *International Journal of Pharmacy Practice*, 2, 86–9.

Smith, F. J. and Salkind, M. R. (1990a). Factors influencing the extent of the pharmacist's advisory role in Greater London. *Pharmaceutical Journal*, 244, R4–R7.

Smith, R. (1997). The future of health care systems: information technology and consumerism will transform health care world wide (editorial). *British Medical Journal*, 315, Saturday 24 May.

Sooman, A. and MacIntyre, S. (1995). Health and perceptions of the local environment in socially constricting neighbourhoods in Glasgow. *Health and Place*, 1, 15–26.

Speckens, A., van Hemert, A. M. and Spinhovel, P. *et al.* (1995). Cognitive behavioural therapy for medically unexplained physical symptoms: a randomised control trial. *British Medical Journal*, 311, 1328–32.

Spiker, P., Anderson, I., Freeman, R. and McGilp, R. (1995). Pathways through psychiatric care: the experience of psychiatric patients. *Health and Social Care in the Community*, 3(6), 343–52.

Stacey, M. (1988). Concepts of health and nature of healing knowledge (1): lay concepts of health and illness. *The Sociology of Health and Healing*. London: Unwin.

Stewart, M., Belle Browne, B., Weston, W., McWhinney, I., McWilliam, C. and Freeman, T. (1995). *Patient-centred Medicine Transforming the Clinical Method*. London: Sage.

Stimson, G. and Webb, B. (1975). *Going to See the Doctor*. London: Routledge.

Stoller, E. P. and Kart, C. (1995). Symptom reporting during physician consultation: results of a health diary study. *Journal of Ageing and Health*, 7(2), 200–32.

Suchman, E. (1964). Sociomedical variation among ethnic groups. *American Journal of Sociology*, 70, 319–31.

Sutters, C. A. and Nathan, A. (1993). The community pharmacist's extended role: GPs' and pharmacists' attitudes towards collaboration. *Journal of Social and Administrative Pharmacy*, 10, 70–84.

Taylor, J. and Gree, M. (1993). NPM consultations: an analysis of pharmacist availability, accessibility and approachability. *Journal of Social and Administrative Pharmacy*, 10, 101–8.

Taylor, J. and Stuveges, L. (1992). Selection of cough, cold and allergy products. Rate of consumer–pharmacist interaction. *Journal of Social and Administrative Pharmacy*, 9, 59–65.

Telles, B. and Pollack, M. (1981). Feeling sick: the experience and legitimation of illness. *Social Science and Medicine*, 15(9), 243–51.

Thomas, D., Absi, E. and Shepherd, J. (1995). The demand for primary dental care at a dental teaching hospital, 1989 and 1993. *Health Trends*, 27(1), 20–22.

Thompson, S., Sobolew-Shubin, A., Galbraith, M., Schwankovsky, L. and Cruzen, D. (1993). Maintaining perceptions of control: finding perceived control in low-control circumstances. *Journal of Personal and Social Psychology* (United States), 64(2), 293–304.

Thorogood, N. (1990). The use of bush amongst Afro-Caribbean women. In N. P. Abbott and G. Payne (eds) *New Directions in Sociology of Health*. London: Falmer Press.

Trogan, A. (1989). Benefits of self-help groups: a survey of 232 members from 65 disease related groups. *Social Science and Medicine*, 29(2), 225–32.

Tuckett, D. (1976). *Introduction to Medical Sociology*. London: Tavistock.

Tully, M. P. and Temple, B. (1997). Who are the people who visit and do not visit pharmacies? A descriptive study, using 'CHAID'. *Pharmaceutical Journal*, 26, 34.

Twaddle, A. and Hessler, R. (1977). *A Sociology of Health*. St Louis, MO: Misby.

Uitenbroek, D., Kerekovsk, A. and Festchreva, N. (1996). Health, lifestyle behaviour and socio-demographic characteristics – a study of Varna, Glasgow and Edinburgh. *Social Science and Medicine*, 43(3), 367–77.

Unell, J. (1986). Supporting self-help in health and social care. *Social Science and Medicine*, 29(2), 245–52.

Vahabi, M. and Ferris, L. (1995). Improving written patient education materials: a review of the evidence. *Health Education Journal*, 54(1), 99–106.

Vallis, J., Wyke, S. and Cunningham-Burley, S. (1997). Users' views and expectations of community pharmacists in a Scottish commuter town. *Pharmaceutical Journal*, 258, 457–60.

Vanagthoven, W. M. and Plomp, H. (1989). The interpretation of self-care – a difference in outlook between clients and home nurses. *Social Science and Medicine*, 29(2), 245–52.

Van Castern, V., Leurquin, P., Baertelds, A., Gurtner, F., Massari, V., Maurice-Tison, S. *et al.* (1993). Demand patterns for HIV-tests in general practice: information collected by sentinel networks in 5 European countries. *European Journal of Epidemiology*, 9(2), 169–75.

Veerhaak, P. F. M. and Tijhuis, M. A. R. (1992). Psychosocial problems in primary care – some results from the Dutch national study of morbidity and interventions in general practice. *Social Science and Medicine*, 35(2), 105–10.

Verbrugge, L. (1984). Health diaries – problems and solutions in study design. In C. Connell and R. Groves (eds) *Health Survey Research Methods*. Rockville: National Centre for Health Services.

Verbrugge, L. (1985). Triggers of symptoms and health care. *Social Science and Medicine*, 20(9), 855–76.

Verbrugge, L. and Ascione, F. (1987). Exploring the iceberg: common symptoms and how people care for them. *Medical Care*, 25: 539.

Vickery, D. M. and Lynch, W. D. (1995). Demand management – enabling patients to use medical care appropriately. *Journal of Occupational and Environmental Medicine*, 37(5), 551–7.

Vickery, D., Golaszewski, E., Wright, E. and Kalmer, H. (1988). The effect of self-care interventions on the use of medical service within a Medicare population. *Medical Care*, 6, 580–8.

Vincent, J. (1992). Self help groups and health care in contemporary Britain. In M. Saks (ed.) *Alternative Medicine in Britain*. Oxford: Clarendon Press.

Virtanen, P. (1994). An epidemic of good health at the workplace. *Sociology of Health and Illness*, 16(3), 394–401.

Vollrath, M., Koch, R. and Angst, I. (1993). Binge eating and weight concerns among young adults from the Zurich cohort study. *British Journal of Psychiatry*, 160, 498–503.

Wadsworth, M., Butterfield, W. and Blaney, R. (1971). *Health and Sickness: The Choice of Treatment*. London: Tavistock.

Waitzkin, H. and Magana, H. (1997). The black box in somatization, unexplained physical symptoms culture and narratives of trauma. *Social Science and Medicine*, 45(6), 811–25.

Waldron, I. (1983). Sex differences in illness incidence, prognosis and mortality: issues and evidence. *Social Science and Medicine*, 17(16), 1107–23.

Walker, R. (1997). Attitudes to over the counter medicines. In *OTC Directory*. London: Pharmaceutical Association of Great Britain.

Walker, R., Macbride, A. and Machan, M. (1977). Social support networks and the crisis of bereavement. *Social Science and Medicine*, 11, 35–41.

Walsh, M. (1995). The health belief model and use of accident and emergency services by the general public. *Journal of Advanced Nursing*, 22(4), 694–9.

Weich, S., Lewis, G. and Mann, A. (1996). Effect of early-life experiences and personality on the reporting of psychosocial distress in general practice – a preliminary investigation. *British Journal of Psychiatry*, 168(1), 116–20.

Wennberg, J. E., Barnes, W. A. and Zubkoff, M. (1982). Professional uncertainty and the problem of Supplier Induced Demand. *Social Science and Medicine*, 16(7), 811–24.

White, K. L., Williams, F., Greenberg, B. G. and Hill, C. (1961). The ecology of medical care. *New England Journal of Medicine*, 265, 885–92.

Whittaker, P., Wilson, R., Bargh, J., Chapman, M. and Dudley, R. (1995). Use and misuse of purchased analgesics with age. *Pharmaceutical Journal*, 254, 553–6.

Wilkin, D., Butler, T. and Coulter, A. (1997). *New Models of Primary Care:*

Developing the Future. A Development and Research Programme. Primary Care Discussion Paper 2. Manchester: National Primary Care Research and Development Centre.

Williams, R. (1983). Concepts of health: an analysis of lay logic. *Sociology*, 17, 2.

Williams, A., Robbins, T. and Sibbald, B. (1997). *Cultural Differences between Medicine and Nursing.* Manchester: National Primary Care Reseach and Development Centre.

Winefield, H. and Murrell, T. (1992). Verbal interactions in general practice, information, a support and doctor satisfaction survey. *Medical Journal of Australia*, 157, 677–82.

Winkler, R., Underwood, P., Fatovitch, B., James, R. and Gray, D. (1989). A clinical trial of a self-care approach to the management of chronic headache in general practice. *Social Science and Medicine*, 29(2), 213–19.

Woloshynowych, M., Valori, R. and Salmon, P. (1998). General Practice patients' beliefs about their symptoms. *British Journal of General Practice*, 48, 885–90.

Wright, P. (1987). The social construction of babyhood: the definition of infant care as a medical problem. In A. Bryman, B. Bylteway, P. Allatt and T. Keil (eds) *Rethinking the Lifestyle.* Basingstoke: Macmillan.

Wyke, S., Hewson, J. and Russell, I. T. (1990). Respiratory illness in children: what makes parents decide to consult? *British Journal of General Practice*, 40, 226–9.

Zadoroznyj, M. and Svarstad, B. L. (1983). Gender, employment and medication use. *Social Science and Medicine*, 31, 225–42.

Zola, I. (1973). Pathways to the doctor: from person to patient. *Social Science and Medicine*, 7, 77–89.

INDEX

HEALTH CARE REFORM
LEARNING FROM INTERNATIONAL EXPERIENCE

Chris Ham (ed.)

If you want a broad introduction to international health care reform, written by some of the best health policy analysts alive today, then this is it.

Chris Heginbotham

- What policies have been adopted to reform health care in Europe and North America?
- Which policies have worked and which have failed?
- What new initiatives are emerging onto the health policy agenda?

This book provides an up-to-date review and analysis of health care reform in five countries: Germany, Sweden, the Netherlands, the United Kingdom and the United States. It reviews the experience of introducing competition into the health service as well as policies to strengthen management and change methods of paying hospitals and doctors. The experience of each country is described by experts from the countries concerned. In this lucid introduction, Chris Ham sets out the context of reform, and in the conclusion identifies the emerging lessons.

The book provides an authoritative introduction to health care reform in Europe and North America at a time of increasing political and public interest in this field. It has been designed for students of social policy and the full range of health service practitioners on courses of professional training.

Contents
The background – The United States – The United Kingdom – Sweden – The Netherlands – Germany – Lessons and conclusions – Index.

Contributors
Reinhard Busse, Chris Ham, Bradford Kirkman-Liff, Clas Rehnberg, Freidrich Wilhelm Scwartz and Wynand van de Ven.

160pp   0 335 19889 9 (Paperback)   0 335 19890 2 (Hardback)